"The Cathedral" by Auguste Rodin (1910)

"did man possess the natural armour of the brutes,
he would no longer work as an artificer, nor protect
himself with a breast-plate, nor fashion a sword
or spear, nor invent a bridle to mount the horse
and hunt the lion. Neither could he follow the
arts of peace, construct the pipe and lyre, erect
houses, place altars, inscribe laws, and through letters
and the ingenuity of the hand, hold communion with
the wisdom of antiquity, at one time to converse with
Plato, at another with Aristotle, or Hippocrates."

GALEN

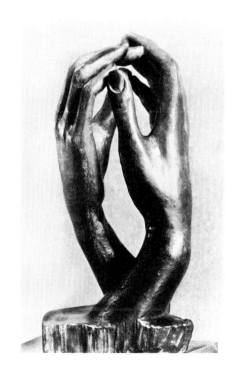

The Hand of "David" (sculptured out of marble by Michelangelo in the early sixteenth century)

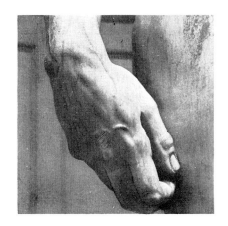

"We ought to define the Hand as belonging exclusively to Man—corresponding in its sensibility and motion to the endowments of his Mind, and especially to that ingenuity which, through means of it, converts the being who is the weakest in natural defense, to be the ruler over animate and inanimate nature. . . ."

SIR CHARLES BELL (1832)

the HAND

as a mirror of systemic disease

THEODORE J. BERRY, M.D., F.A.C.P.

Instructor in Medicine,
University of Pennsylvania School of Medicine;
Staff Physician, Pennsylvania Hospital,
Lankenau Hospital, and Bryn Mawr Hospital

 F. A. DAVIS COMPANY · *Publishers* · Philadelphia

To my children—

Candy

David

Jeff

Becky

Thad

with my appreciation for their tolerance

Preface

A careful examination of a patient's hand may supply the physician with a great deal of useful information. When a patient becomes aware of the physician's interest in his hand the usual reaction is one of quizzical amusement and the inevitable question follows: "What can you tell by looking at my hand?" This book represents a clinician's effort to outline what might be seen in the hand in a wide variety of pathologic and physiologic states.

I recall many years ago, while I was in the early primary grades at school, it was the custom of the school doctor to make periodic visits for the purpose of examining the pupils. His examination consisted of the briefest of surveys during which the tongue, throat, and hands were inspected. The children were lined up and marched past the physician, who stood in front of the classroom by a window. The queue shuffled hurriedly along in a rough semblance of order with palms turned up, fingers spread wide, and tongues stuck well out. Having thus devoted something on the order of a few seconds to each child, and apparently satisfied with the results of his hasty scrutiny, the doctor departed ceremoniously. A question lingers in mind until this day: Was the nameless apostle of Apollo uncommonly astute or simply (and more likely) a pitiable slave of Time?

There may be a moral here: If given a short interval in which to deduce as many facts of clinical significance as possible, a trained inspection of hands is an excellent way to begin, for a careful study of this magnificent member of the human body may provide an incredible amount of useful data to the physician who is willing to exploit his powers of observation. It is possible that the Mohammedans held a similar view since at one time it was their custom to limit the exposure of their women during a medical interview to the hand alone, thrust modestly through a parted curtain.

General facts and broad impressions as well as data of pathologic interest can be accrued by examining the hand. These may aid materially in a better understanding of the individual as a whole. The expressive hands of the orator, the dancer, or the actor contribute as generously to the broader effect of his performance as do his mannerisms of speech, movement, or facial expression. Aptitudes and certain traits of personality, temperament, and emotional reserves are revealed in the configuration, gestures, and use of a person's hands. These characteristics are apparent even when the individual is not engaged in his usual occupation or activities. Stigmas of adaptive changes in the hands produced by work or play testify to the kind of usage through the presence of stains and calluses or by signs of wear or of muscular development. Some concept of the maneuverability and dexterity of the hands, suggesting to the examiner certain occupational or intellectual potentials, can be assessed even during their quiet distracted activity.

A physician's first contact with the patient offers a visual over-all appraisal. This long-view introductory inspection should be augmented by the most traditional custom of greeting—a handshake. By this means, some degree of mutual assessment is at once possible. A general impression of temperament or personality of the individual is transmitted and the physician may benefit by observing the temperature, texture and moisture of the skin, and the muscular tone and vigor, size and configuration of the hand. Of course, the same opportunity for evaluation is available to the patient as well, and he may draw his own impressions of the physician at the same time the physician is making his appraisal of the patient, enhancing or diminishing the patient's confidence and rapport.

Mannerisms and affect are amplified by the conduct of the patient's hands, his facial expressions, and the way he delivers a verbal account of his symptoms, all of which contribute to the total clinical evaluation. An observant clinician can assign diagnostic importance to the way a patient uses his hands to locate or describe a painful symptom. The individual with peptic ulcer, for example, may point with one finger to the right of the mid-epigastrium. Spasms of hollow organs are frequently described by the sufferer by clenching the fist and pressing it against the abdominal wall at the appropriate area. The pain of coronary artery disease is usually described by its victim by drawing the fingertips of both outspread hands across the chest from a starting point at the midsternal line. Or such a patient may lay his palm flat against the middle of his sternum and press against his chest. The diagnosis of the common tension headache is sometimes made possible by observing the patient spread the fingers of one hand across his brow with his thumb on one temple and the remainder of his hand spanning across his eyes as one might do to shade them from the light. Or he may cup his hand at the nape of his neck just below the occiput.

Such adjunctives to a general physical impression are available for evaluation by the observant examiner who will accept the advantage of every possible parameter in his clinical appraisal. No organ or anatomic structure other than the hand or any laboratory procedure can reveal so readily so much practical information about the patient as can the hand; nor is there any other structure so convenient and accessible for examination.

In an effort to stimulate interest in more precise diagnostic perception among the house officers and medical students, my colleagues and I have contrived a game of detection at the bedside that has met with gratifying enthusiasm and some degree of success as a tool for instruction. The object of the challenge is to attempt to draw as many facts that relate to the clinical problem under investigation as possible by means of a thorough inspection of the patient. This inspection is unaided by palpation, percussion, or the use of any diagnostic implements of any kind. After all the data have been collected from this source of information, the remainder of the physical examination is completed. Primarily for academic purposes, the fostering of the importance of the physical examination requires a reciprocal de-emphasis of reliance upon the laboratory and roentgenographic studies. Consequently, the student is allowed eventually to augment his findings and impressions made on physical examination by whatever special laboratory procedures he considers likely to be most informative, the expenditure for the procedure to be minimal, an arbitrary and imaginary sum of money being designated.

During these exercises it soon became apparent that a close inspection of the hands gives a greater wealth of information of clinical importance than does similar scrutiny of any other part of the body.

I believe that every physician derives unconscionable pleasure in solving the unknown or clarifying the obscure. Doubtlessly, Dr. Arthur Conan Doyle, the renowned physician-author, experienced vicarious satisfaction from his characterization of this principle in the prototype of the master detective, Sherlock Holmes. By employment of deductive reasoning, Holmes developed his case study largely by intensive inspection. It is believed that the character of Holmes was fashioned after one of the great and colorful physical diagnosticians of that age in the British Isles, Sir Joseph Bell, one of Dr. Doyle's real-life heroes.

In generations past, physicians developed keen skills in the interpretation of morphologic changes in their patients. Deprived as they were of our modern laboratory methods and special diagnostic procedures such as the x-ray examination, electrocardiography, and the employment of isotopic techniques, their compensating excellence in methods of physical diagnosis was an art born of necessity.

In approaching the project of compiling data on the hand relating to clinical medicine, one is impressed by the voluminous material which has accumulated on the subject over many centuries. Numerous obvious temptations to stray along philosophic tangents are avoided with reluctance. I have, however, attempted to adhere firmly to the prime purpose of this monograph—the presentation of a simple outline of several manifestations of morphologic or functional effects in the hand which are associated with systemic diseases.

Its intimate participation in the hazards of an active environment renders the hand particularly susceptible to injuries of one kind or another. In fact, the hand is more often the site of trauma than is any other part of the body. Various surgical techniques arising out of the need to repair and rehabilitate the injured hand require special consideration but are out of context with my more limited purpose. There are extant several excellent surgical treatises devoted to the management of traumatic defects and the correction of congenital anomalies of the hand. Excluded from the book by the same criteria are the dermatologic lesions which involve the hand only as it represents a portion of the total skin. Congenital malformations which have no particular bearing on the various internal systems have been similarly excluded.

It seems totally unnecessary to champion the argument for the economic importance of the hand when one considers the magnitude of a person's economic limitations if hand function is impaired or lacking. Certain employment opportunities are available to leg amputees and the sightless, but it tests the imagination to suggest a type of gainful occupation for the unfortunate individual with uncompensated loss of hand function. It has been estimated by a research group that the hand performs approximately 1000 different functions in an ordinary day's activity. The thumb participates in almost all of these functions—a fact which clearly makes it the most important of all digits.

The use of the hand has contributed largely to man's rise above the lower animals, and has developed to such a high level of utility largely through the existence of a thumb capable of opposing with the fingers, a feat not achieved by any other primate. During the earliest years of life the human being learns of the outside world by use of these specialized grasping and exploring antennae. Experience gained by such exploration allows for the development of a basic intelligence which subsequently provides motivation for these same hands throughout life. The manner and proficiency of utilization and the degree of sensory capacity of the hands vary greatly among individuals, depending upon the person's inborn tendencies and acquired skills and the physical forces brought to bear on the hands. Each individual thus possesses his own personal pattern of hand development. These patterns of movement and expression are as characteristic of the owner as is his face or posture.

The human hand, incredibly endowed with fineness of movement and capacity for close obedience to the eye and mind, has made possible many of man's skills and arts. Painters and sculptors have stressed the beauties, strength, and artistic expressivity of the hand in the portrayal of mood or personality of their subjects. Emphasis on the hand in art appears in the works of Michelangelo, Leonardo da Vinci, Rodin, and many other masters. The mood and emotional content of a painting or other work of art is so often portrayed in the execution of the hands that this representation forms a most important medium of expression in art.

Apparently, man has focused his attention on the hand long before there were written historical records. That the hand has had extended significance as an art form and religious symbol is well documented. In use today are countless expressions of hand language—customary gestures, salutes, signals, and symbols—which bring to our own time an extension of ancient recognition of the hand's importance as a means of communication. Gestures and hand signs may project mental images which successfully overcome language barriers and often transcend limits of vocal communication. An articulate speaker develops the judicious use of the power of accentuated speech through use of his hands. Quintilian, the fabled instructor of public speaking, made reference to the orator's hands nineteen centuries ago: "For other parts of the body assist the speaker, but these I may say, speak for themselves."

Many ancient philosophers pondered the teleologic implications of the human hand and debated the cause-and-effect relationship in the hand's development and the emergence of man's intellect. Aristotle and Pliny engaged in lengthy disputes during their search for the answer as to whether the development of the hand was causally related to the improvement of the intellect, or whether the intellect was responsible for the hand's evolution. Anaxagoras was adamant in his belief that "man's superiority is owing to his hands." Aristotle contended that the hand was "the organ of organs, the active agent of the passive powers of the entire system."

Less altruistic in their application of shrewd observation are the colorful charlatans and palm readers who have constructed traditional tribal monopolies throughout the ages. On more objective analysis, the mechanics of their chiromantic trade is based on a blend of common sense and remunerative stagecraft. Even a slanting reference to the collected lore on the subject would fill many volumes and transgress beyond the boundaries of this prospectus.

I have collected the following material freely from the experience and work of many other observers, but withal the catalogue does not presume to be complete—rather, it represents a loose under-structure upon which the reader interested in this useful adjunct to diagnosis may be enticed to add further data.

It is a fervent hope that the approach to this outline of systemic mechanisms which are capable of producing physical effects in the hand will generate a renewed interest in closer inspection and attention to the obvious, and provoke a stronger development of a waning bedside art—fuller use of the powers of observation.

THEODORE J. BERRY

Acknowledgements

The collection of photographs and other data on the hand as it mirrors internal disease began as a tiny trickle many years ago. Then its mass reached a level where my own personal observations were limited by time and availability of clinical material. I had originally attempted to collect photographs to demonstrate each of the disease entities for the purpose of completing the teaching catalogue of possibilities. Obviously, such an attempt represented a startling inaccuracy of judgment, as has been discovered by so many others who have attempted to exhaust a topic of trivia. Incompleteness is inescapable. I borrowed the thoughts, observations, and pictures of many widely scattered authors to add to my own material whenever possible. But still the saturation point is far off and the thirst of acquisition common to all collectors continues short of satiety.

I would like to say that I have personally observed each clinical entity described in this book. However, in order to bridge wide gaps in the outline, it was necessary to augment experience with material exotic to the locale of my own observations. And I doubt that I shall ever have the opportunity to photograph the hands of a patient with pinta or with leishmaniasis.

It would be an herculean task to list all those who have been willing or unwitting accomplices to this work, but a brief litany of "without whom's" seems justified.

First, I owe my public expression of gratitude to my dear wife whose art work adorns this book literally from cover to cover, its effectiveness lying bare for the reader's own evaluation. What is more obscure, however, is this lady's immeasurable patience in the art of dealing with an impatient part-time author. I am indebted to a similarly tolerant secretary, Miss Lillian Consalvi, and to Mrs. Muriel Lewis, who typed and retyped without murmuring. Dr. Perry S. MacNeal allowed me to select illustrations from the fine collection of teaching Kodachromes on file at the Pennsylvania Hospital, most of which he had photographed himself. Dr. Raymond Krain contributed several excellent photographs and helped tremendously by giving advice from the dermatologist's viewpoint. I had the advantage of the counsel of two outstanding authors, Dr. William B. Bean and Dr. F. Dennette Adams, who read the early drafts of the manuscript. Dr. Robert Bower offered useful technical advice on the final draft. W. Robert Swartz deserves thanks for his capable photofinishing work and conversion of my slides to reproducible prints.

The friendly and helpful assistance offered me by the F. A. Davis Company, particularly by Mr. R. Kenneth Bussy and Mrs. Patricia Reichenbach, has been a gratifying experience.

To the many scores of similarly inquisitive physicians who have contributed to the general fund of medical knowledge, to my own teachers and colleagues, and most of all to the students of medicine who display such fresh interest and avidity for the "pearls" in the study of our Art, I extend my everlasting indebtedness and thanks.

And finally, with special gratitude, I wish to express my appreciation to Dr. Edward L. Bortz, who first conceived the possibilities of a monograph from a highly disorganized assortment of material. As time went by, it was he who insisted that I draw an end at this arbitrary point. The pregnancy had gone long enough—and reluctantly I permitted induction of labor, for better or worse.

T. J. B.

Table of Contents

3 Diseases of the Nervous System

1

disorders of the ENDOCRINE SYSTEM

It is interesting to reflect upon the numerous instances in which the form and function of the hand are related to disorders of the endocrine system. Psychologic disturbances, and those diseases affecting the nervous system, are perhaps the next most commonly encountered clinical situations which are associated with predictable physical effects in the hands. To syllogize, this linkage of glandular and behavioral disorders may not conflict seriously with reason when one considers the broad common-ground that exists between them. In many clinical entities which affect the endocrine system a concomitant psychic disturbance is also present. Occasionally the emotional disorder assumes major importance taking symptomatic precedence over the primary disease. For example, the commonly encountered "premenstrual tension syndrome" embraces a variety of electrolyte and bodily water effects which are secondary to hormonal imbalances, and which characteristically produce indisputable psychic phenomena. Other combined effects of a similar relationship are to be noted in the dramatic and unfortunate postpartum psychosis, or in the lesser-order neurosis termed so colorfully by the laity "the lying-in blues."

Thyroid hormonal disorders, either "too much" or "too little," are attended by psychologic symptoms if the "nervousness" of the hyperthyroid state qualifies. "Myxedematous madness," an unforgettable alliterative expression, refers to the psychotic effects sometimes observed in hypothyroidism.

The effects of temperament and emotional patterns that are attributed to the menopausal syndrome range from annoying, low-

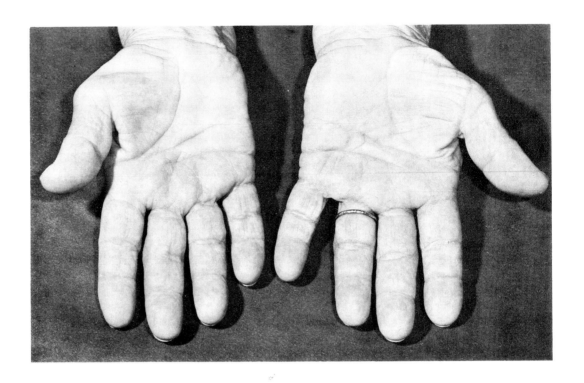

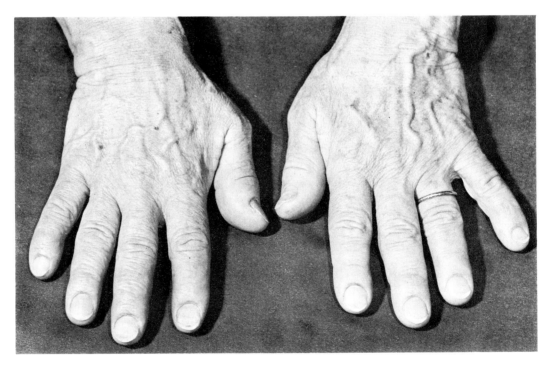

Fig. 1. Acromegaly. *Upper*, Spade-hand configuration, palmar view. *Lower*, Dorsal view; note spoon-nail deformity of the index and middle fingers, right hand.

grade depressions to major psychotic episodes with mental deterioration.

In many instances the specific diagnosis of a glandular disorder may be suggested to the examiner at the first study of the configuration of the hand structure, particularly in the shape and size of the hand, and the proportions of the fingers, the texture, temperature, and color of the skin, and the moisture content of the palms.*

The endocrinologist, more so perhaps than any other specialist among the divisions of clinical medicine, can employ with greater accuracy the principles of diagnosis by simple, skilled inspection.

ACROMEGALY

Tumorous involvement, or functional hypertrophy of the anterior pituitary gland, excites such dramatic morphologic changes in the patient's gross bodily appearance that the diagnosis is frequently possible on these criteria alone. The hand participates in a predictable manner as part of the over-all characteristic transition to gigantism and consequent generalized coarsening of many of the anatomic landmarks.

Classically, acromegaly first appears in the third decade of life. The early changes involve an enlargement of the head, hands, and feet, and bitemporal hemianopsia and headache. Skeletal surface exaggerations occur, leading to the development of the characteristic "horse-face," owing to prominence of the jaw, and bony ridges in the head and face, and kyphosis and lordosis.

The hand becomes elongated and broadened, is coarse and swollen-looking, and an exaggeration of its outline occurs that has caused it to be likened to a spade ("spade-hand"). The various planes of the palm are blocked out in geometric masses bordered by deeply set creases. The fingers appear stolid and stodgy and lack the normal tapering at the tips. Consequently, dexterity is diminished and mobility and graceful movements are lost. The nails are broadened and have quadrangular tips, but do not demonstrate any abnormal curving or clubbing. Spoon-nail deformity and occasionally simple nail-plate hypertrophy occur in acromegaly.

PITUITARY INSUFFICIENCY

When pituitary function is insufficient as a result of either developmental arrest, or as a sequel to apoplectic catastrophe or other destructive process, the hand may demonstrate a physical configura-

* Werner describes "nine endocrine hand types" in his text, Endocrinology (1942).

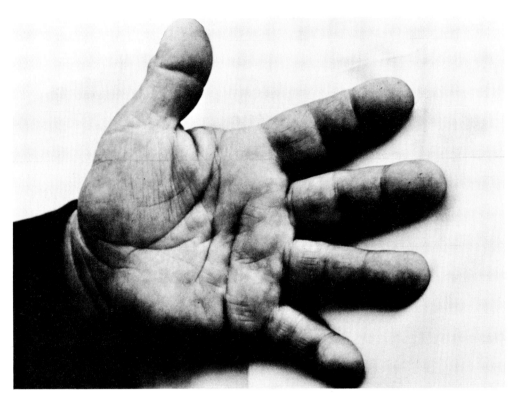

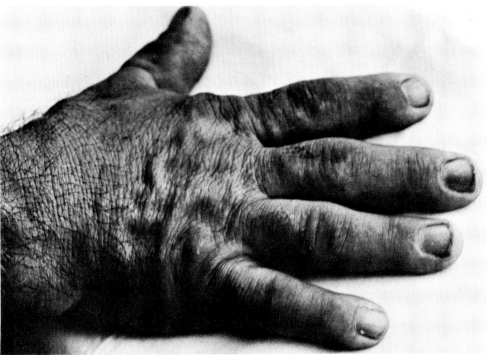

Fig. 2. Acromegaly. Palmar and dorsal views of "spade-hand" configuration; broad, thick, pudgy hand. Note deep creases and coarse, sausage-shaped fingers.

tion of a characteristic nature. Usually the phalanges are long and slender, with tapering ends, and the palm and wrist are narrow. The over-all appearance suggests a weakness or delicacy of movement, although specific tests of motor strength are not necessarily abnormal. In many ways the hand of the patient with pituitary insufficiency is directly opposite in form to that of the patient with acromegaly.

In pituitary infantilism the individual is well-proportioned but diminutive, like the famed Tom Thumb of the old circus. The hands are appropriately small, but perfectly formed.

PITUITARY OBESITY

The bones of the hand are representative of long bones elsewhere in the body. Epiphyseal closure takes place at the proper time, or is early or delayed, in the same manner and degree as the other long bones under similar hormonal influences, so that delayed closure of the epiphyses due to endocrinopathic mechanisms will cause morphologic changes in the appearance of the hand that conform to the over-all build of the person. Generally, the configuration of the hand is characteristic for the specific glandular abnormality, although, like many clinical entities, gradations and sub-types exist, and combinations of endocrine defects may occur in the same individual.

The type of hand seen in patients with various endocrine disorders will depend in part upon whether the disease preceded or followed the attainment of normal adult growth.

There are two types of pituitary obesity—the juvenile and the adult. The hands in juvenile pituitary obesity are short, fat, and pudgy, with fingers that are either tapered or pointed. The proximal phalanges are sausage-shaped and are much shorter proportionately than is the long, soft, squarish palm. There is a characteristic padding of fat on the dorsal surface of the hands and on the proximal and middle phalanges. The distal phalanx does not exhibit such padding and, consequently, appears slender or relatively tapered.

A high degree of flexibility in the fingers permits the terminal phalanges to be bent farther backward than normal, so that most often these patients are said to be "double jointed." Musculature in the palms is poorly developed, and although the palms are relatively large the greater bulk is made up of fatty tissue rather than muscle.

In the adult form of pituitary obesity the shape of the hand is determined by the time of onset of the disorder. If the patient had the disease as a child there is a carryover of the same type of hand as in the juvenile subject. Another adult type of pituitary obesity occurs after bone maturation has taken place. Such an individual

Fig. 3. Pituitary obesity. Short, fat, pudgy hand and tapered fingertips in the juvenile form of pituitary obesity. This subject's hand demonstrates a childlike, chubby softness which belies his age (22 years) and size (265 pounds).

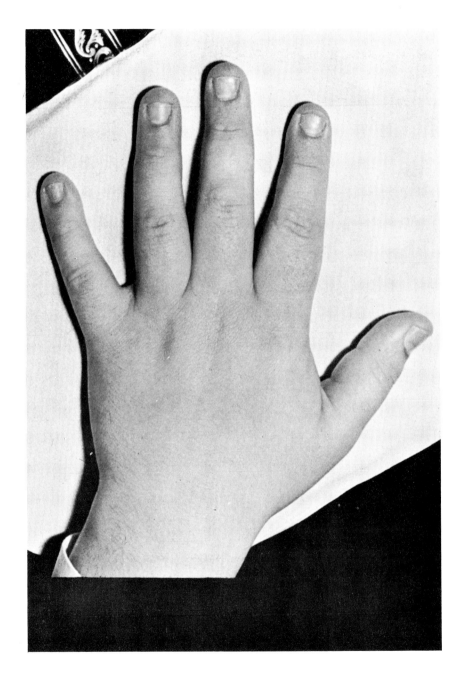

gains weight rapidly, particularly in the girdle area, but the hands and face do not become fat. Dorsal padding on the hand and first two phalanges does not occur. Neither are the fingertips tapered.

HYPERTHYROIDISM

The hand of the patient with hyperthyroidism is never cold. This statement is a break with an ancient aphorism that outlaws the use of the words "never" and "always" in the language of Medicine, but so far in our experience it has endured inviolate.

In hyperthyroidism the hands are often long and bony, with thin fingers, especially the basal phalanx. In these respects they resemble the classically slender hands of the tuberculous patient. The nails are often long, shiny and curved, and, because of hypermetabolic effects, have an increased growth rate. The skin of the hand is characteristically smooth and satiny, and moisture of the palm is usually excessive. A fine tremor of the hand is accentuated by forceful extension and spreading of the fingers, but is not readily distinguishable from the nonspecific tremor seen in the tense, anxious individual or the rather coarse trembling that occurs not infrequently as an isolated familial trait.

The warm, wet hand of the hyperthyroid individual is in sharp contrast with the cold, wet hand found in the neurocirculatory asthenic, and the differentiation is an important point in the diagnosis. Emotional stress and anxiety are capable of producing an excessive palmar perspiration which can sometimes assume symptomatic proportions. Such a condition may interfere with the proper use of the hands engaged in particularly fine occupational maneuvers. Many patients, under the stress of a medical consultation, will be embarrassed by an uncontrollable perspiration, particularly prominent in the hands. Observation of this evident trait cannot help but impart some information about the patient's temperament to the examiner.

Clubbing of the fingers, and isolated enlargement of the phalanges have been noted in patients with severe exophthalmos. These states occur rather rarely and the condition is termed "thyroid acropachy." The second and third phalanges become thickened bilaterally, and the phenomenon is reportedly related to the development of a hypothyroid state after treatment of hyperthyroidism. Its development has been found to take place from six weeks to seven years after therapy for hyperthyroidism.

The toes may be clubbed as well, and sometimes subperiostial new bone formation is noted in the metacarpals and phalanges, with tufting of the terminal phalanges. A suggested explanation of this

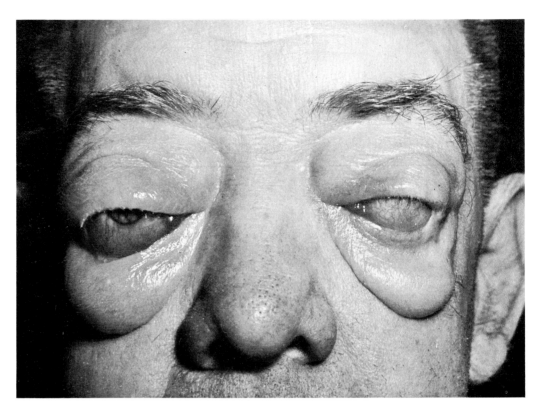

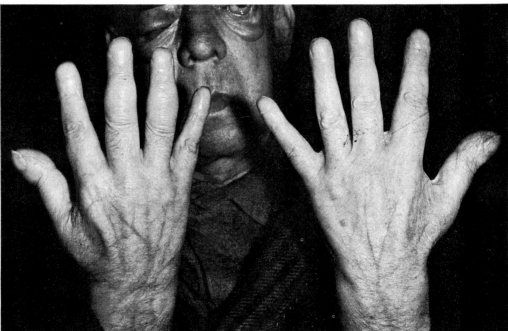

Fig. 4 A & B. Thyroid acropachy. Isolated enlargement of the phalanges in a patient with malignant exophthalmos. This deformity has been noted as a delayed effect of the hypothyroid state which follows treatment of hyperthyroidism. (Courtesy of Raymond Greene, M.D.)

Fig. 5. Adult myxedema. A, Note characteristic facies and dry, puffy hand of a patient with myxedema, and B, the changes that occur after treatment with thyroid extract. (Courtesy of Lisser and Escamilla: Atlas of Endocrinology. C. V. Mosby Co.)

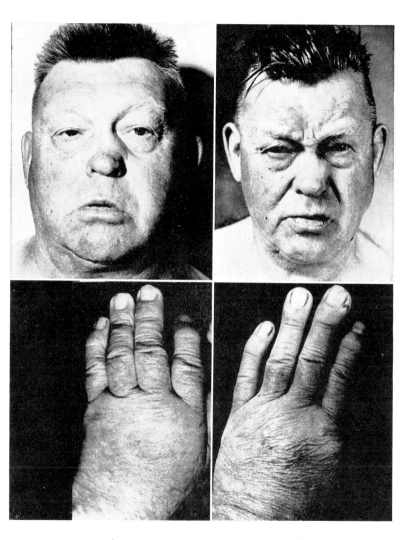

A　　　　　　　　B

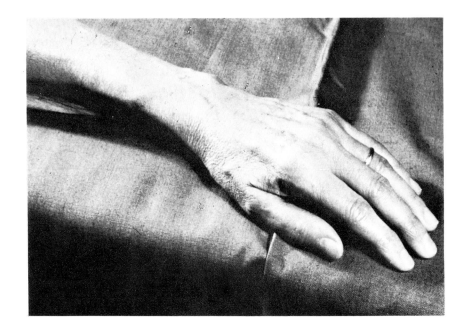

Fig. 6. Addison's disease. Diffuse pigmentation, especially marked over the knuckles.

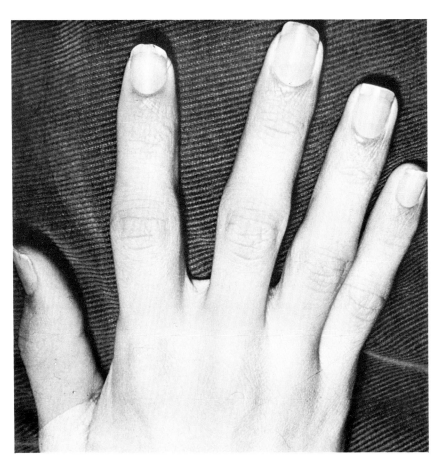

Fig. 7. Addison's disease. Note faint rim of pigmentation of the skin in the nail fold just proximal to the nails.

phenomenon, not completely acceptable, is that it represents an alteration in vascular dynamics of bone, owing to the sudden change in peripheral blood flow when hyperthyroidism is replaced by the hypothyroid state. However, in a single reported instance of thyroid acropachy, exophthalmos was unassociated with a known prior state of thyrotoxicosis.

Another effect of hyperthyroidism observed in the hand is the occasional finding of thickening and vertical ridging of the nails in patients long afflicted with this disease. This physical abnormality and others, such as brittleness or loosening of the distal ends of the nails, may occur in either hypothyroidism or hyperthyroidism.

HYPOTHYROIDISM

When myxedema is fully developed it is seldom difficult to detect its presence on general physical examination in the course of which the classic sleepy, pudgy, expressionless, pallid face is quickly recognized. The hand participates in the general hypometabolic status and has a characteristic doughy, dry, rough feel and stolid appearance. The palms are pale and sallow and in some instances a distinct hyperkeratosis is noted. When the onset of the defect has antedated full bodily maturation and growth of the individual, the hands are short and stubby with sharply tapering fingers. The hand appears larger than normal and flatter in the hypothyroid individual. The nails often become brittle and demonstrate retardation of growth, sometimes showing the "spoon-nail" deformity (koilonychia).

A non-pitting type of edema may often be observed in hypothyroidism, and occasionally xanthomatous infiltrations in the skin of the fingers occur, reflecting the presence of hypercholesterolemia in this disease. Other nail-plate deformities, such as atrophy and psoriatic-like pitting, may be observed.

ADDISON'S DISEASE

Adrenal cortical insufficiency of sufficient duration and magnitude may be associated with electrolyte imbalance and increased cutaneous pigmentation. The latter effects are demonstrated in the hand by a generalized, coppery, pigment deposition in the skin. This usually appears earliest about the knuckles, and seldom involves the palms, except in the creases where it is particularly pronounced. Extremely dark brown, almost black, freckles are found over the dorsum of the hand and elsewhere on the exposed surfaces of the

Fig. 8. Clubbing and telescopy
of distal phalanges in patient with
hyperparathyroidism. Control normal right hand. (Courtesy of
Escamilla: Laboratory Tests in
the Diagnosis and Investigation
of Endocrine Functions. F. A.
Davis Co.)

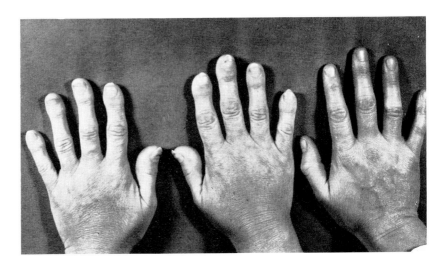

Fig. 8

Fig. 9. Hyperparathyroidism.
A form of clubbing occurs in hyperparathyroidism owing to resorption of bone at the distal
phalanges. Note thinning of the
end phalanx and partial disappearance of the tufts. (Courtesy of
Lisser and Escamilla: Atlas Endocrinology. C. V. Mosby Co.)

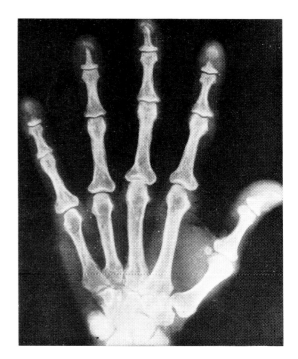

Fig. 9

body. The fingernails frequently appear darker than is normal—usually some shade of yellow.

Sun-tanning, in richly pigmented, asthenic, but otherwise normal individuals, poses a diagnostic challenge, so that gross inspection requires additional avenues of study to establish an adrenal origin when Addison's disease is suspected.

CRETINISM

Cretinism is associated with a pronounced underdevelopment of the hand both functionally and morphologically.

The hand of the cretin is usually broad and very short with stout fingers and spatulate tips. The fifth finger is undersized, pointed and crooked, a variation which is frequently noted in individuals of retarded physical or intellectual development. The thumb is ugly and misshapen, being quite shortened, and has a blunted bulbous terminal phalanx. Nail development is poor and striations are common. Overgrowth of the cuticle (pterygium) further obscures the lunulae, which are either rudimentary or absent. The palms and fingers are covered with a dry, cold, hard and pallid, inelastic skin which gives an excessive rigidity and torpidity to the feel and movements of the hand. These same characteristics are noted in practically all of the various congenital developmental disturbances, including such conditions as cerebral palsy, or other dystrophic abnormalities. When intellect and mental maturation are for any reason retarded or obtunded, the defect is usually paralleled in the development of the hand, as related to both function and form. The hand of the mentally or physically retarded patient usually lacks muscular tone as well as graceful and fine movements. The use of the fingers is partially limited to awkward mass maneuvers rather than each digit having individuality or purposeful action. Thumb strength may be impaired and the major functions of this digit are often ineffectual.

HYPERPARATHYROIDISM

Functioning adenomas of the parathyroid gland produce certain classic clinical features such as hypercalcemia, a characteristic dryness of the mouth, increased thirst, renal colic, skeletal deformities and a tendency to peptic ulceration. Less prominent in the clinical constellation is the development of clubbed fingers. The ends of the fingers may display a bulbous formation due to resorptive effects of disease at the distal phalanges.

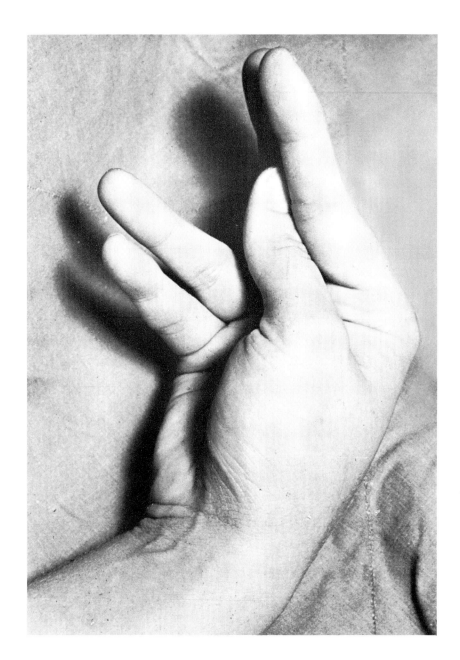

Fig. 10. Carpopedal tetany in hypoparathyroidism. Similar spasms of the wrist and fingers occur in numerous clinical conditions accompanied by hypocalcemia or alkalosis.

HYPOPARATHYROIDISM

Parathyroid disorders, whether due to the presence of a functioning adenoma or to the diminished availability of the parathyroid hormone, exert their physiologic effects largely through disturbances of calcium and phosphorus metabolism. The osseous and dermal organs are particularly affected, so that diagnosis is suggested first by the physical appearance of the patient, who has dry, scaly skin, unusual pigmentation and abnormally sparse hair distribution. Confirmation of this impression is made by the laboratory study of the calcium-phosphorus relationships and roentgen-ray examination of the skeletal system.

Perhaps also related to calcium imbalance, hypoparathyroid states may be associated with changes in the appearance of the fingernails. Atrophy and a psoriatic-like pitting of the nail plates may occur. The normal surface contour is lost and wavy crinkling of the nail edge develops. This effect is a part of a generalized cutaneous disorder in which the hair becomes sparse and the skin is dry and pigmented.

Inadvertent removal of the parathyroid glands during thyroidectomy is the foremost cause for the production of hypoparathyroidism. Muscular irritability, due to the lowered ionizable calcium concentrations in the serum, and a development of the dramatic phenomenon, carpopedal spasm, are early clinical manifestations of this effect.

CARPOPEDAL SPASM ("Accoucheur's Hand" or "Obstetrical Hand")

Carpopedal spasm may be considered at this point in connection with hypoparathyroidism, although it may occur in any of the many other pathophysiologic situations in which the level of serum ionizable calcium is sufficiently depressed. At approximately 3.5 milliequivalents per hundred milliliters a critical serum calcium concentration is reached below which tetanic manifestations usually occur. During an attack of tetanic spasm the hand assumes a characteristic posture in which there is a bilateral flexion of the fingers at the metacarpophalangeal joints while the phalanges are extended. The thumbs are drawn almost to the little finger, the wrists are slightly flexed and there is slight ulnar deviation. An attack can be provoked during quiescent intervals by production of venous stasis by means of a tourniquet applied to the forearm (Trousseau's sign).

Hypocalcemic tetany and carpopedal spasm may occur in a number of other clinical conditions. A partial list includes: (1) hyperventilation alkalosis, (2) uremia, (3) nephritis, (4) nephrosis, (5) rickets, (6) sprue; malabsorption syndrome, (7) pregnancy; lactation, (8) osteomalacia, (9) protracted vomiting; pyloric obstruction, (10) alkali poisoning, (11) toxicity to certain drugs (morphine, lead, alcohol, etc.).

BRACHYMETACARPALIA
(Associated with Pseudohypoparathyroidism and Pseudopseudohypoparathyroidism)

The term "brachymetacarpalia" is applied to an abnormal shortening of the metacarpals, which occurs predominantly in the fourth and fifth metacarpals and is occasionally found in association with pseudohypoparathyroidism and pseudopseudohypoparathyroidism. In both of these curious disturbances with classically cumbersome titles, the patient appears short and stubby of form generally, with a rounded face and faulty hair development, and presents areas of ectopic calcification and brachymetacarpalia.

Brachymetacarpalia can be demonstrated best by having the patient make a fist, and by observance of poorly developed, or absent, fifth or both fourth and fifth knuckles. The nails are often short and broad. Mental deficiencies of varying degrees are frequently associated.

Pseudohypoparathyroidism represents a target organ defect rather than a primary parathyroid gland abnormality, but since a calcium-phosphorus imbalance occurs a consequent susceptibility to hypocalcemic tetany exists. This disorder, also known as the Seabright-Bantam syndrome, presents the same clinical picture of chemical disturbances and physical characteristics as are found in the hypoparathyroid patient, although there is no lack of available parathyroid hormone, but rather an inability to respond to parathormone.

Since the patient with pseudopseudohypoparathyroidism represents no chemical abnormality, but displays only the physical appearance of the other two conditions, tetany does not occur.

When the clinician is alerted to this association, careful examination of the hands of the patient afflicted with tetanic seizures and who is found to have short, broad nails and absent fourth and fifth knuckles in the closed fist, a diagnosis may be made which spares the individual a needless survey in the epileptic clinic.

SYMPTOM OF DU BOIS

Hand shape follows a genetic pattern. We have observed a shortened fifth finger and fifth metacarpal in females of three generations. No other defect, such as abnormal calcium-phosphorus levels in the blood serum, or the stigmata of pseudopseudohypoparathyroid habitus, could be detected in these individuals.

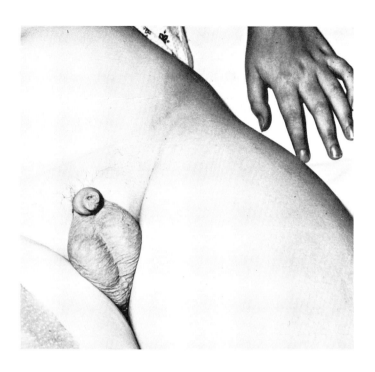

Fig. 11. Fröhlich's adiposogenitalis dystrophy. Note the soft, fat, dimpled hand and tapered fingers in a teen-age subject with underdeveloped genitalia.

Fig. 12. Preadolescent eunuchoidism. Female, age 31 years, whose eunuchoid state was present before puberty, demonstrates the characteristic narrow wrist and long, non-tapered fingers. (Courtesy of Lisser and Escamilla: Atlas of Endocrinology. C. V. Mosby Co.)

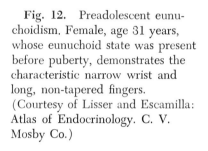

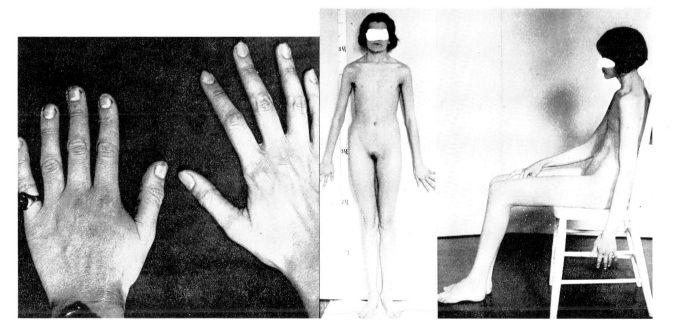

FROHLICH'S DYSTROPHY ADIPOSOGENITALIS

The diagnosis of Fröhlich's dystrophy adiposogenitalis is usually strongly suggested to the examiner by the physical appearance of the individual. The classic distribution of obesity through the girdle area and the presence of genital hypoplasia are well known. Abundant deposits of fat in the breasts and mons veneris are characteristic.

Acromicria, a small, broad hand, is another associated outstanding physical trait.

The patient afflicted with this endocrine disorder usually has smoothly textured fingers with broad bases, which extend from dimpled knuckles and taper sharply to slender tips. The small, relatively delicate hand contrasts strikingly with the generalized soft obesity of the trunk.

HYPOGENITALISM

Doubtlessly gonadal development is closely correlated with the general configuration and growth of the hand.

Two types of hands are recognizable among eunuchoid individuals. One type is quite fat, and this variety is more often seen in men than in women, the hands being soft-skinned, weak in appearance and in their movements, and quite pale. The pallor of the castrate's hand is replaced by the normal pink color when testosterone is administered to the patient. The other type is the thin, elongated hand which is more often seen in women. Both the palms and fingers are slender and graceful, with long nails curved in an exaggerated way from side to side and having big moons. Exceptional flexibility in the palm, and in the fingers particularly, and the delicacy of posturing and gesturing bestow on the hand the elegant air which suggests the fine hand of the artist. The castrate's fingernails are frequently ridged, thickened and heaped up to suggest oyster-shell arrangement (onychauxis).

2
disorders of CONNECTIVE TISSUE

Grouping of several apparently diversified diseases into a category labeled "dyscollagenoses" has certain advantages to clinicians both from a diagnostic and a therapeutic standpoint. Membership in this classification has been limited to those disorders with a common target organ, the mesenchymal layer of the embryo. Listed among the collagen diseases are such conditions as rheumatoid arthritis, rheumatic fever, systemic lupus erythematosus, serum sickness, scleroderma, and dermatomyositis. As time passes it is possible that additional pathophysiologic entities will be reoriented into this classification, to include psoriasis, the carpal tunnel syndrome, Dupuytren's contracture and others.

The common denominator is connective tissue involvement by swelling, nodularity or change in density. Most of these diseases affect the small joints by thickening, or are characterized by inflammatory swelling of periarticular tissues, muscles, tendons, ground substance, or other fibroblastic structures.

Because of its histologic composition a fertile soil for such changes is present in the hand. Many of the arthritides and dyscollagenoses are manifested early and progressively in the digital or carpal articulations and their associated fibrous supporting materials. And because of characteristic anatomic features, such as the rich network of sensory nerves and highly precise motor functions, minimal degrees of inflammatory interference are promptly appreciated, objectively and subjectively.

Other systemic diseases of connective tissue which either primarily

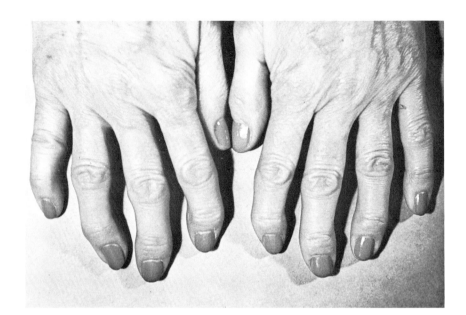

Fig. 13. Osteoarthritis. Angulation deformity of the distal phalanges; the thumbs are usually spared.

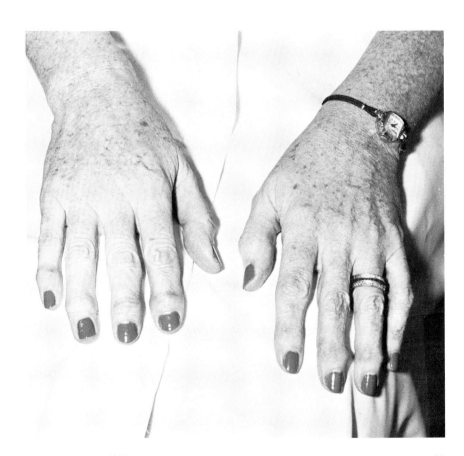

Fig. 14. Osteoarthritis. Painful Heberden's nodes on all fingers except the thumbs.

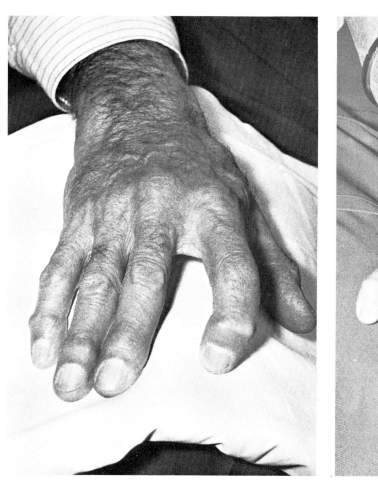 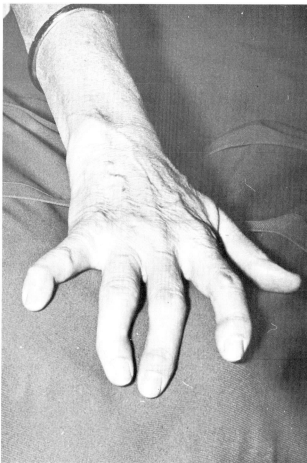

Fig. 15   Fig. 16

Fig. 15.   Osteoarthritis. Heberden's nodes at the distal interphangeal joints.

Fig. 16.   Osteoarthritis. Characteristic nodule formation at the distal joints (Heberden's nodes) and angulation of the terminal phalanges. Note the relatively normal thumbs.

or incidentally produce physical or functional alterations in the joints frequently cause signs in the hands. Some of these diseases and several collagen disorders are included in this chapter.

OSTEOARTHRITIS

Perhaps the most common systemic disturbance that is seen in the hand is osteoarthritis, or degenerative arthritis. It has been estimated that approximately 5 per cent of all persons over 40 years of age in this country will have symptoms, and as high as 90 per cent of individuals in this age group display roentgen-ray evidence of the process. The cartilages of the distal finger joints are usually the first to show the effects of wear and tear, although the weight-bearing joints are theoretically more susceptible to traumatic effects. Women are afflicted much oftener than men (about 10 to 1) and there seems to be an increased incidence among overweight people.

Small knobs develop at the distal ends of the middle phalanges (Heberden's nodes). These nodules are cartilaginous and bony enlargements which are frequently associated with flexion and lateral deviation deformity. They may appear singly but more often are multiple. Most commonly they appear at the ends of the middle phalanx of the index and middle fingers, but only very rarely are the thumbs involved. These nodes are sometimes accentuated by additional swelling due to superimposition of superficial synovial cysts filled with a clear gelatinous material. Heberden's nodes are transmitted genetically as a recessive trait in the male, and as a dominant one in the female.

In contrast with rheumatoid arthritis, in which the middle phalangeal and the metacarpophalangeal joints are most often involved, osteoarthritis classically begins at the distal finger joints, and only later may extend to include the middle phalangeal and the metacarpophalangeal joints as well. Lateral deviation of the distal phalanx and tenderness of the fingers create an annoying, painful disability in a large percentage of the older female population.

RHEUMATOID ARTHRITIS

Some of the earliest manifestations of rheumatoid arthritis occur in the hands. Initially, such changes are confined chiefly to the proximal interphalangeal joints, which become thickened symmetrically and produce a spindle-form or fusiform appearance to the digits. As the disease progresses a combination of flexion deformities and dislocations occurs. Later, ankylosis causes characteristic crippling dysfunction and a physical appearance familiar to all clinicians.

Fig. 17. Rheumatoid arthritis. Early spindling of the digital joints, which are periodically tender and painful.

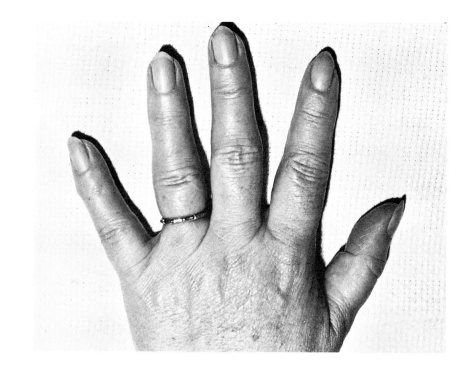

Fig. 18. Rheumatoid arthritis. Of all the damaging effects in the hand which are the result of rheumatoid arthritis, extension deformity is perhaps the most serious because it interferes with the gripping function. Note also the dusky fingertips and the irregular, dystrophic nails.

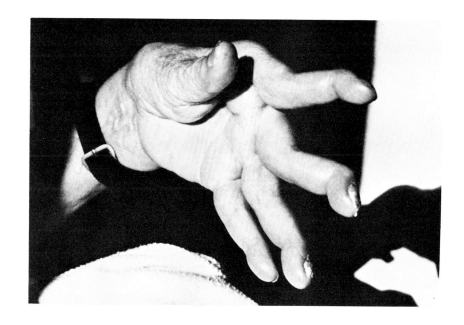

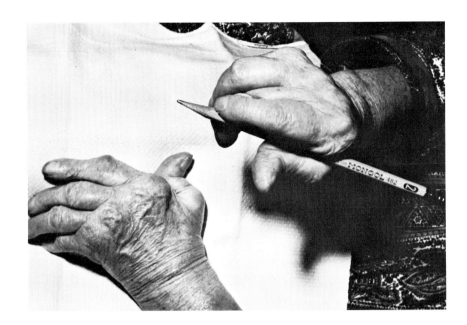

Fig. 19. Rheumatoid arthritis. There is tendon dislocation and subluxation of distal phalanx of the thumb. Sharp angulation of the tip interferes seriously with many of the thumb functions such as picking up small objects and manipulation of a writing or other implement. This patient has compensated for her defect by a grip on the pencil which is characteristic in patients with rheumatoid arthritis.

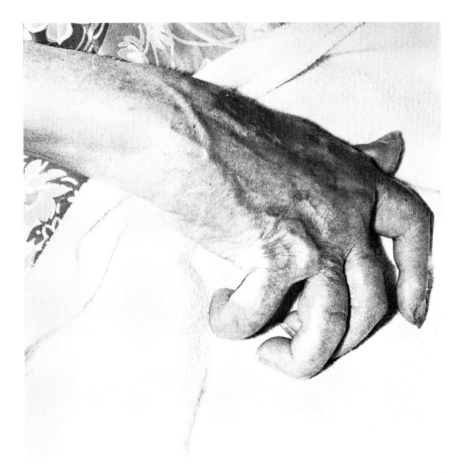

Fig. 20. Rheumatoid arthritis. Extension deformity in the left hand, ulnar deviation and dislocated extensor tendon in fifth finger of the right hand. Note also the trophic changes of the fingernails.

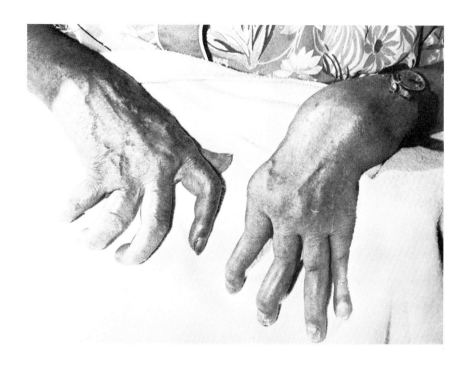

Fig. 21. Rheumatoid arthritis. Note large dorsal synovial cyst and atrophic changes in the adductor muscles of the thumb. Metacarpophalangeal joints are swollen and stiff.

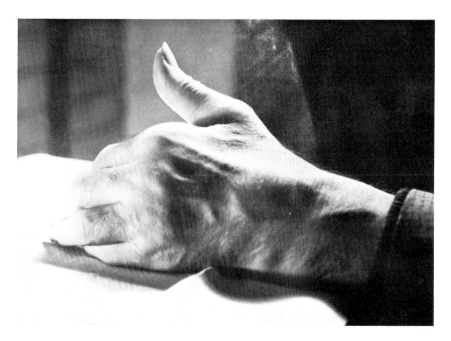

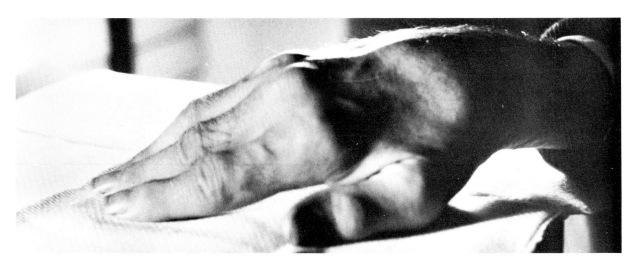

Fig. 22A.   Rheumatoid arthritis. Note maximum involvement of the metacarpophalangeal joints, lesser involvement of the middle digital joints, and normal distal joints. This contrasts with the order usually seen in osteoarthritis.

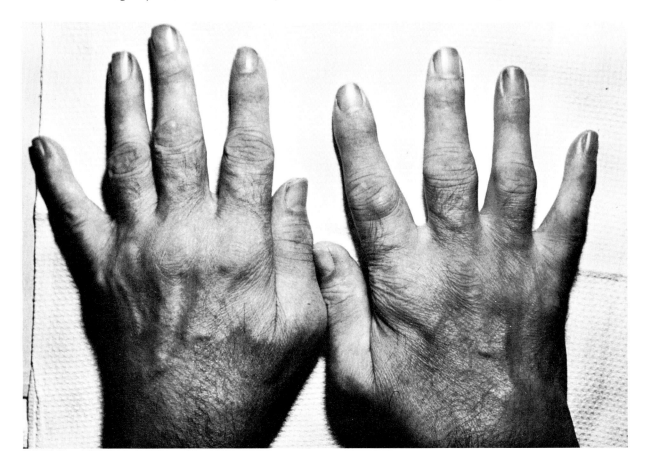

Fig. 22B.   Rheumatoid arthritis. Note enlargement of the metacarpophalangeal joints and the middle phalangeal joints. Distal joints are spared. A ganglion is present on the right index finger, just proximal to the middle joint.

Although the disease as it presents in the hands is particularly disposed to affect the metacarpophalangeal and middle phalangeal joints, the distal phalangeal joints may become involved subsequently. This sequence of progression contrasts with degenerative arthritis, in which condition the earliest changes usually involve the distal digital joints, and only later include the proximal joints.

The earlier stage of active inflammation in the joints, tendons and intrinsic muscles is replaced later by more permanent deformities. These include ulnar deviation of the fingers, which is often associated with anterior subluxation or lateral dislocation of the joints and extensor tendons. The exact cause for ulnar deviation remains obscure, and although this particular deformity is quite commonly noted to occur in the hands of individuals with rheumatoid arthritis, the principal problem is a cosmetic rather than a functional one. The greatest degree of digital deviation is found in the fifth finger, and lessens stepwise toward the radial side, the least effect being in the index finger. The defect is accentuated by a frequently associated pre-existent dislocation of the digital tendons.

Of all the disabling deformities produced in the hands by rheumatoid arthritis, the type which creates the highest level of functional impairment is due to fixation of the digits in hyperextension. By seriously interfering with proper gripping function the hand is rendered virtually useless.

Multiple rheumatic nodules may develop in the subcutaneous and periarticular tissues. The nodules range in size from a millimeter in diameter up to 2 or 3 centimeters. They are firm, sometimes tender, and occur most frequently in or adjacent to tendons of the metacarpophalangeal joints and on the dorsal aspect of the index and middle fingers. Small, tender rheumatoid nodules may be observed in the palmar surfaces of the tendon sheaths of proximal phalanges. Thickening and stiffness of the wrist produce a wooden character to the movements of the hand and consequently seriously diminish dexterity.

Atrophy of the interossei muscles and the thenar pad occurs from disuse and permits an overpull of unaffected muscles. Shortening of the fingers results, and skin folds appear in unusual places. If the distal phalanx is grasped and pulled axially, the over-riding phalanges can be extended to normal length, which accounts for the term, "opera glass hand," applied to this type of deformity. Severe degrees of involvement may eventuate in complete ankylosis and grotesque configurations which may create the appearance of crowded, gnarled fingers, atrophic musculature and a variety of degrees of distortion familiar to all physicians.

Alternating stretching and destruction of periarticular tissues may

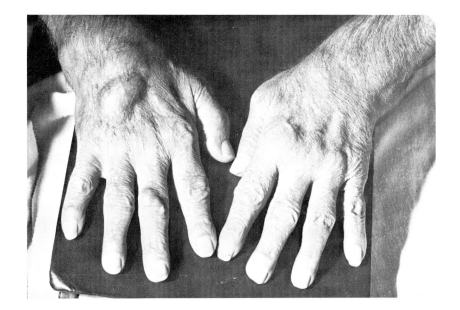

Fig. 23. Rheumatoid arthritis. Note synovial cyst on the dorsum of the right hand in a patient with rheumatoid arthritis.

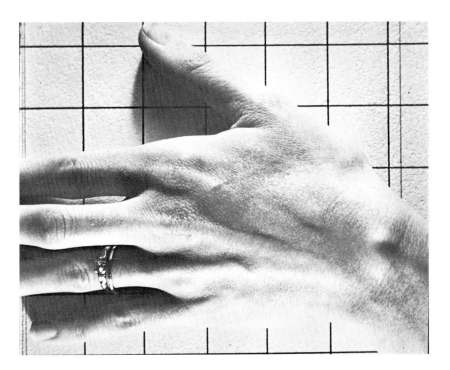

Fig. 24. Simple ganglion of the wrist.

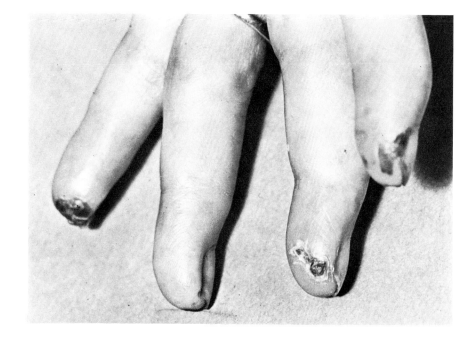

Fig. 25. Arteritis in rheumatoid arthritis. Gangrene of the fingertips due to arteritis complicating rheumatoid arthritis. (Courtesy of Sir John Richardson, St. Thomas Hospital.)

Fig. 26. Mallet finger.

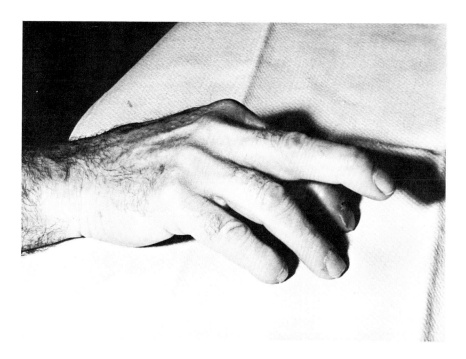

produce increased mobility in the joints in any direction, abetted by rupture of the ligaments and subluxation or dislocation of joints. Tendons, too, may become dislocated, stretched or ruptured. Weakness and contracture deformities of the intrinsic muscles of the hand occur. Through a combination of any or all of these mechanisms a wide variety of abnormalities may be incurred.

Sometimes large ganglions or synovial cysts are formed, especially on the dorsum of the hand and about the wrist. These are fibrous walled cysts, with single or multiple chambers which contain a water-clear gelatinous material and fluid in varying proportions. The larger ones are fluctuant on fingertip ballottement. When ganglions increase in size they may cause further mechanical interference with hand function, but are seldom tender except when they have exceeded the limits of skin and local tissue elasticity.

Frequently a defect in thumb function is encountered in rheumatoid arthritis, in which capacity for rotation becomes impaired. When the thumb cannot rotate properly the patient is unable to pick up small objects. When rotation is inadequate the sensitive fleshy pad of the thumb fails to make contact with the opposing digit and fine movements are thereby hindered. In other instances the thumb may be unstable laterally and this causes a serious fault in the integrity of the grip.

Rupture of extensor tendons may occur; this may be either complete or incomplete, producing a "mallet-finger" deformity. Occasionally a "trigger-finger" deformity may be observed in patients with rheumatoid arthritis. Under such conditions, flexion of the finger is normal, but active extension may be impossible. The finger can be straightened only passively by the other hand. Small fibrous masses and thickened areas form on the surfaces of tendons. These interfere with the smooth sliding movement under the transverse palmar bands which encircle the tendons.

There are several other systemic diseases which are associated with arthritic manifestations—sarcoidosis, systemic lupus erythematosus, ulcerative colitis, psoriasis, rubella, etc., all of which may demonstrate joint swelling and deformity similar, morphologically, to the changes observed in rheumatoid arthritis.

PSORIASIS

Psoriasis is a commonly encountered multi-system disease. The findings on examination of the hand may be all that is required to arrive at the diagnosis. The characteristic cutaneous lesion is usually located on the extensor surfaces of the body, particularly involving skin overlying the joints. The rash of psoriasis is a dry, white or light

Fig. 27. Psoriatic arthritis. Involvement of the joints with arthritic enlargement, irregularity of the nails and characteristic skin rash on both hand and foot.

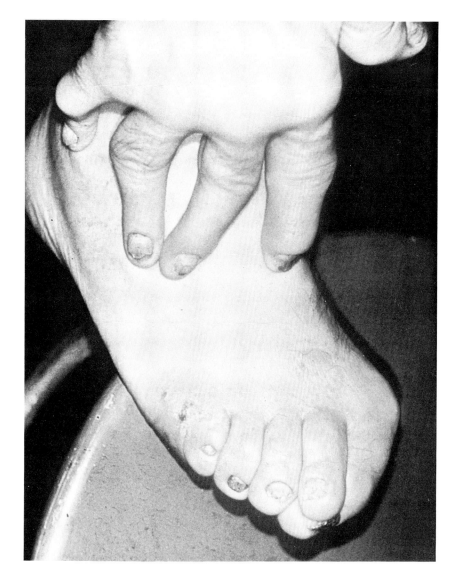

Fig. 28. Psoriasis. Deeply pitted thumbnail in psoriasis.

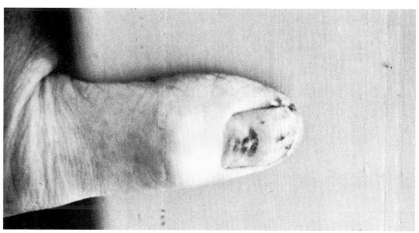

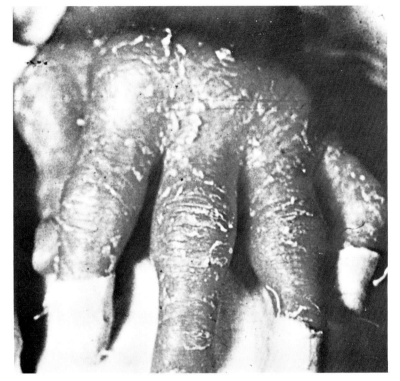

Fig. 29. Psoriasis. A, Skin, joint and fingernail involvement. B, X-ray film of thumb joint showing destruction by psoriatic arthritis. C, Irregular nail, thickened, arthritic distal thumb joint and scaling skin rash of psoriasis.

A

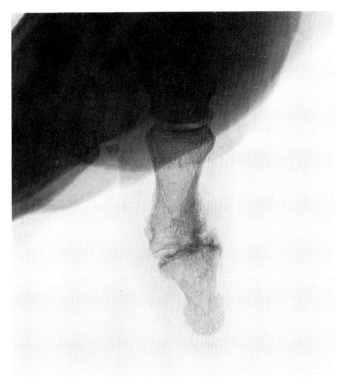

B

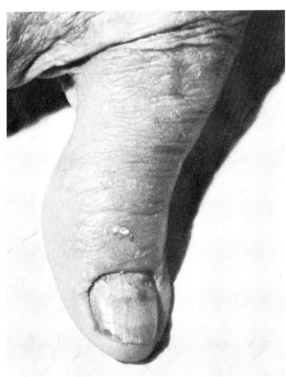

C

gray scale irregularly covering a dull red, sharply outlined base. Periarticular swelling is noted in the hand, usually at the distal phalangeal joints. The nails are thickened or irregular and show small shallow pits. Subungual chalky deposits may form and honeycombing of the nail plates may occur.

Arthralgia is intermittent, as are the cutaneous effects. Favorable response appears to follow ultraviolet or solar irradiation, and, more recently, remission has been reported following adrenocortical steroid therapy. Winter weather and emotional or physical stresses seem to worsen the entire symptom complex. Other disorders, especially metabolic or nutritional defects, are frequently associated with psoriasis. These include hepatic nutritional cirrhosis, diabetes mellitus, gout and chronic alcoholism. Many psoriatic patients have overt psychoneurotic tendencies which closely parallel the cutaneous rash.

The thumb of the patient with psoriasis may demonstrate all of the cardinal physical manifestations of the disease: the distorted, enlarged and sometimes tender distal joints, the oyster-shelled and pitted nail plates, and the characteristic silvery-scaled red rash on the knuckles.

In the differential diagnosis, mycotic infection of the nails and gouty arthritis must be considered.

SHOULDER-HAND SYNDROME*

The various liberal uses of the term "shoulder-hand syndrome" have resulted in the definition of a clinical syndrome with an exceptionally elastic boundary. For the purposes of our discussion the concept will be limited to reflex dystrophic disturbances of the extremity which are related to certain internal lesions.

A profusion of inflammatory, neoplastic, cardiovascular and vasomotor disturbances are capable of producing sympathetic dystrophic changes in the upper extremity. Common usage has more narrowly defined the syndrome to involvement of the shoulder and hand with pain and trophic changes following myocardial infarction (post-infarctional sclerodactylia). However, the swollen hand of osteoarthritis and vasomotor disturbances and edema in the paralyzed hand of hemiplegics are also included within the scope of this terminology.

The shoulder-hand syndrome is sometimes associated with more remote pathologic processes, with more obscure teleologic connec-

---

* This entity is not new. As long ago as 1897, Sir William Osler commented on a form of "motor disability" in the shoulder as a sequel to "anginal attacks."

Fig. 30. Shoulder-hand syndrome. Cool, stiff hand in an elderly male patient with carcinoma of the cardiac end of the stomach and extension into the esophagus. The patient is attempting to spread and extend his fingers.

Fig. 31 A-C. Shoulder-hand syndrome. Demonstrating the defect in movement of fingers which produces an incompletely extended hand and an imperfect grip. (Courtesy of Steinbrocker and Argyros: Med. Clin. N. America.)

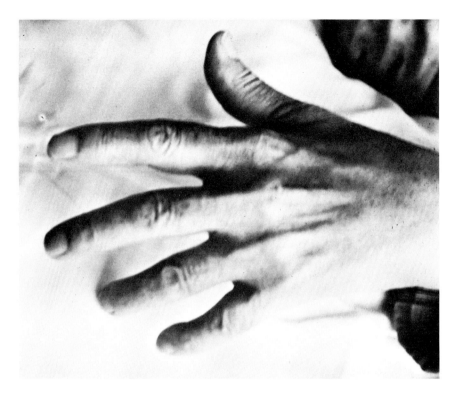

Fig. 30

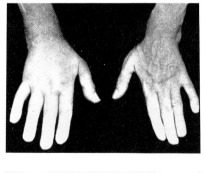
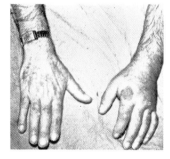
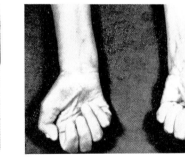
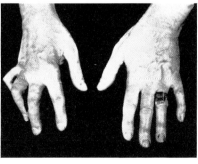
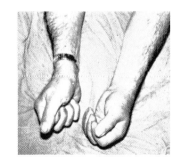
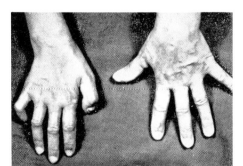

Fig. 31A   Fig. 31B   Fig. 31C

tions, such as, in certain instances, following herpes zoster. Dystrophies in the shoulder and hand muscles occur frequently after calcific tendonitis or peritendonitis of the shoulder, the pain of the inflammatory condition causing limitation of motion and consequent atrophy of disuse.

The superior thoracic sulcus tumor, or the so-called Pancoast tumor, has been related causally to the development of the shoulder-hand syndrome. So also have certain tumors of the brain. My colleagues and I have observed an instance in which painful swelling of the hand and motor disability of the shoulder appeared to be related to intrathoracic extension of carcinoma of the cardiac end of the stomach.

Other mechanisms responsible for the development of the shoulder-hand syndrome include: discogenic disease of the cervical spine, other mechanical impairments which interfere with the vascular supply to the upper extremity (spondylosis, spurring or "lipping" of vertebral bodies), and inflammatory states which involve vessels in the neck, axilla or upper extremity (febrile panniculitis).

Clinically, the shoulder-hand syndrome occurs most frequently in the elderly, most patients being over 50 years of age, and a slight majority of the cases are noted in women. Pain and diffuse tenderness are early symptoms in this syndrome. Cutaneous hyperesthesia and gradually increasing swelling of the hand develop early in its course. The skin is usually dry, cool and inelastic. Movements of the hand are wooden and restricted, particularly noticeable on attempts to extend the fingers. Later, a second stage evolves which is characterized by induration of the cutis and subcutis. Eventually, subtle transition to a state of persistent pain develops, with residual dystrophy progressing sometimes to the formation of contractures. The patient may be unable to extend and spread his fingers, but if any digits are spared the thumb and index finger are most commonly unaffected.

The pain of this disorder usually appears first in the shoulder and represents a classic example of true referred pain. In those instances when it occurs as a sequela of myocardial infarction, it generally appears as early as a week or as late as seven months after infarction. Vasomotor changes which affect the color and temperature of the skin of the hand follow a progressive pattern which begins with blushing or reddening of the skin, and later is replaced by cyanosis or pallor. As the defect advances, the skin of the hand becomes smooth, glossy and cold, and there may be irreversible contractures of the fingers.

Occasionally a type of fascial thickening is observed in the palmar aponeurosis, similar to that seen in Dupuytren's contracture. Physical signs may be unilateral or bilateral, but when only one side is involved the left is more frequently affected than the right. With contractures of the flexor tendons at the wrists and in the digits, a steadily progressive atrophy of the intrinsic musculature occurs. The sweat mechanisms in the skin are often disturbed. Limitation of motion is generally encountered in the metacarpophalangeal and interphalangeal joints.

The shoulder-hand syndrome has been reported to occur in 5 to 20 per cent of patients who have had myocardial infarction. More recently, the incidence seems to be growing less, perhaps as a result of a growing tendency to liberalize the rigid restrictions of activity in the management of myocardial infarction.

One wonders whether the subacromial bursitis, and the painful shoulder seen so frequently after coronary artery occlusion, and frequently among hospitalized patients who are confined to bed, could possibly be caused by the unaccustomed and increased use of the arms in bedfast individuals.

DUPUYTREN'S CONTRACTURE

Dupuytren's contracture is a fibrous thickening and contraction of the palmar aponeurosis which often involves the tendonous extensions to the fingers. Its description is included among the connective tissue diseases, and, although its exact etiologic basis is not clear, there are certain features which suggest placement with the dyscollagenoses.

The earliest lesions are thought to arise from the walls of the small arteries in the palmar fascia. Grossly, the contracture begins with the formation of a tight, hard nodule beneath the skin of the palm at the base of the fourth or fifth finger. As it slowly progresses the overlying skin is dimpled and dense cords form which extend into the palmar aspects of the involved fingers. The fingers are drawn gradually into greater and greater degrees of flexion. In severe cases the tips of the fingers may be flexed until they meet the palm making extension impossible and resulting in serious impairment of hand function. Ankylosis of the associated joints is often a concomitant event. The knuckle pads over the middle joints of the fingers are frequently thickened and resemble the structures normally exhibited in the same location in apes.

Dupuytren's contracture may affect one or both hands, but when it is unilateral the right hand is involved twice as frequently as the left. It occurs in 1 to 2 per cent of the adult population and affects the foot as well as the hand in about 5 per cent. According to published reports, men are seven to ten times more likely than women

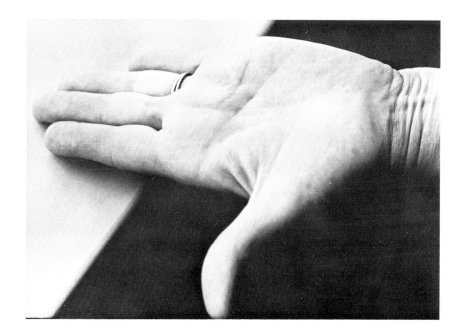

Fig. 32. Dupuytren's contracture. Dimpling of palmar skin; forced extension of the fingers in this early stage of the involvement causes tenseness and blanching of the skin in the proximal phalanx of the fourth finger.

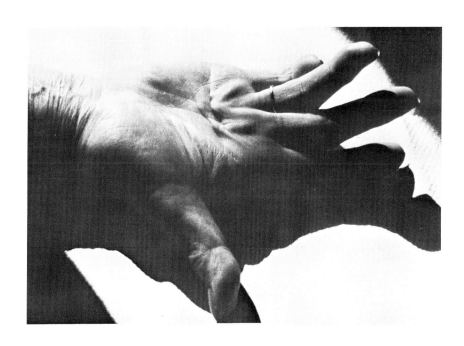

Fig. 33. Dupuytren's contracture. Palmar fascial thickening, dimpling of the skin of the palm and contraction of the ring finger in a patient with hepatic cirrhosis.

to have this condition, although such a wide difference in sex incidence has not been impressive in our experience. An age-linked reference is apparent, older persons being more often affected than the younger ones.

Although the contracture most commonly involves the fibrous extensions of the fourth finger, it may also include any of the other fingers. In order of descending frequency, the fifth, third, index finger and thumb may show Dupuytren's contracture.

There is an hereditary pattern noted in many instances. In the older literature it was suggested that Dupuytren's contracture was an effect related to repeated small traumas incurred in manual laborers, but the theory of such causative associations is no longer considered acceptable. The condition is frequently found in individuals who have contractures elsewhere, such as in Peyronie's disease, and in persons who have a general rheumatic tendency or over-all bodily stiffness.

Dupuytren's contracture has been observed in association with osteoarthritis and certain other systemic diseases such as alcoholic hepatic cirrhosis, diabetes mellitus, gout, psoriasis, and epilepsy. Wegmann reports that 28 per cent of epileptics had palmar fascial fibrosis and 12 per cent showed definite Dupuytren's contracture. The defect appears to be related also to spinal compression syndromes, RH-factor disturbances and tuberculosis.

Wegmann noted an increased incidence in alcoholics with hepatic cirrhosis and parotid hypertrophy (66 per cent) and postulated that fibrosis of the pancreas and the fibroplastic process in the palmar aponeurosis may have a common etiologic factor in alcoholism.

One may wonder whether a hormonal factor may not play a part in the formation of Dupuytren's contracture. The frequency with which this deformity is present in menopausal women, cirrhotic individuals, diabetics, and in certain apparently well subjects who also display palmar erythema underlies this query.

SCLERODERMA

An important early clue in the diagnosis of this dramatic dyscollagenosis is present in the hand. The effects of scleroderma in the hand are due to fibrosis which produces circulatory embarrassment and consequent trophic changes.

At first, the involved skin becomes thickened, and, as induration progresses, the cuticular and subcutaneous tissues become adherent to the underlying structures. The hard, inelastic skin impairs mobility and flexibility, and the hands have a tight appearance that suggests investment in a glove that is too small a size. The skin of the

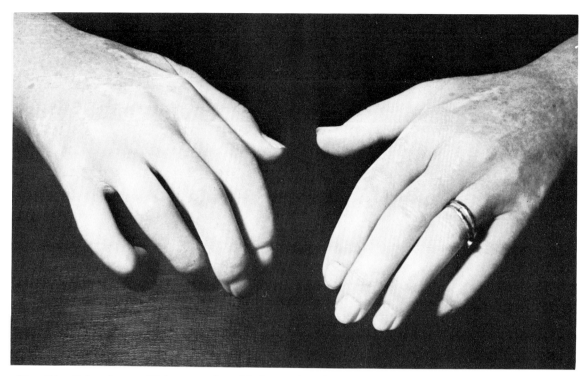

Fig. 34. Scleroderma. Tight, smooth, cold skin and early contractures of fingers in early scleroderma.

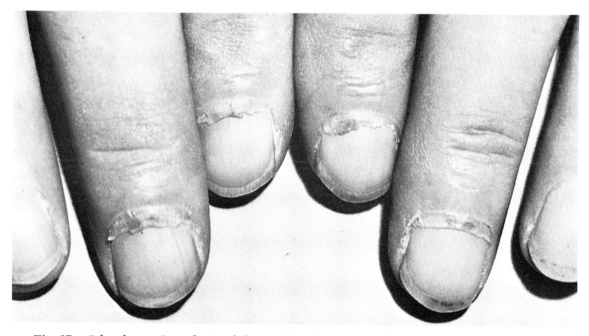

Fig. 35. Scleroderma. Irregularity of the cuticle and pterygium formation occur in many vasospastic disorders such as seen in these fingers of a patient with scleroderma. Small thromboses are present around the nails. (Courtesy of Sir John Richardson, St. Thomas Hospital.)

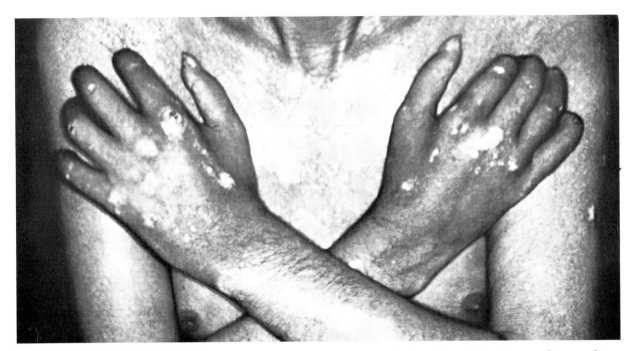

Fig. 36. Scleroderma. Dense white scars of healed ulcerations over the knuckles; tight pigmented waxy skin; curved drawn digits; dystrophic skin and nails.

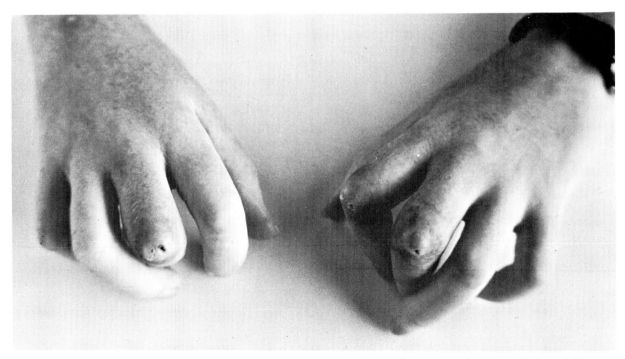

Fig. 37. Scleroderma. Note ulcerations on dorsum of knuckles; absence of creases in the skin and clawed fingers.

fingers appears waxy, and the digital creases are ironed out or altogether lacking. Fixation of the skin diminishes dexterity and fine movements of the fingers. Eventually the digits are drawn into a tense, poorly functioning claw. When these changes produce uncompensated circulatory deficits, especially on the dorsal surfaces of the joints, trophic ulcerations and fissures develop. Circulatory interference may proceed to ultimate stages of gangrene and autoamputation.

Raynaud's phenomenon in the fingers is a common event in the prodromal period. Localized hair loss in involved parts is related to trophic alterations. Cutaneous pigmentation may be either increased or decreased in scleroderma, but more often a diffuse yellowish-brown coloration or mottling of affected skin is observed.

Some writers refer to a "special form" of scleroderma which starts with Raynaud's phenomenon and advances progressively to absorption of phalanges. This condition has been termed "sclerodactylia" or "acrosclerosis," but classification as a separate disease does not seem justified.

Deposits of calcium salts occur rather commonly in the skin, subcutis and muscles throughout the body, especially in the fingers. The high incidence of calcinosis in scleroderma supports the argument that calcium-phosphorus relationships play an important etiologic role. However, the question as to the exact position of calcium metabolism in the pathogenesis of scleroderma has not been answered satisfactorily to date.

In scleroderma the presence of dysphagia, or other evidences of esophageal derangement, and pulmonary insufficiency helps to differentiate the condition from a more benign familial disorder. The latter is transmitted as a dominant genetic characteristic through several members of a family, and is limited to findings in the skin of the hands, which is the locus of a developmental defect in elastic connective tissue.

Occasionally, scleroderma exists concurrently with rheumatoid arthritis, and scleroderma-like swellings of the fingers are seen sometimes in psoriatic arthritis.

POLYMYOSITIS AND DERMATOMYOSITIS

Polymyositis is associated with degeneration and inflammation in and around skeletal muscles and is particularly disposed to affect the proximal limb and girdle musculature. The term "dermatomyositis" is applied to a form of polymyositis in which skin involvement is present. There is a close resemblance of these conditions with others in the connective tissue group, such as rheumatoid arthritis

Fig. 38. Dermatomyositis. The erythematous rash of dermatomyositis, when present, is confined to the skin overlying the knuckles. This distribution contrasts with that observed in systemic lupus erythematosus in which the erythematous involvement extends proximally along the line of the extensor tendons on the back of the hand. (Courtesy of J. Haserick, M.D., Cleveland Clinic, Cleveland, Ohio.)

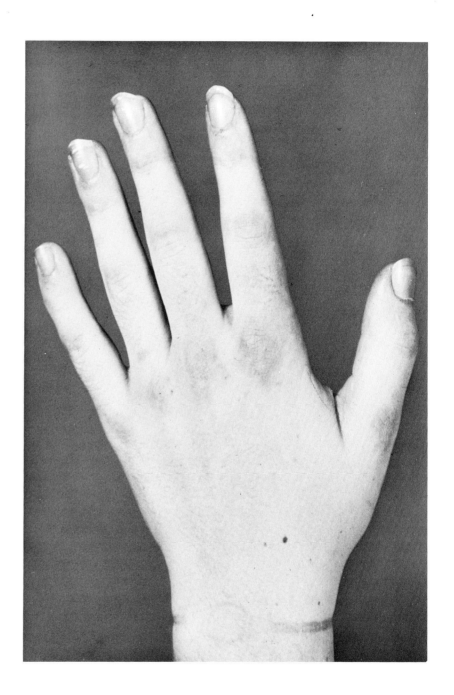

and scleroderma. Diagnosis of dermatomyositis carries additional significance in that there is frequently an associated occult visceral malignant lesion, usually a carcinoma. The commonest sites are the female pelvic organs, breast, lung and colon.

The clinical picture is extremely variable, although muscular weakness of proximal muscles is outstanding. Dermatomyositis often has an acute onset and frequently attacks children, although the relationship with internal neoplasms is more often observed among adult patients. The incidence of malignant disease in dermatomyositis in persons over 40 years of age is near 50 per cent and about 18 per cent in the over-all group.

In about 65 per cent of patients with polymyositis, skin manifestations are present. Dermal effects include a dusky erythema of the face, upper trunk and arms. A heliotrope suffusion of the upper eyelids is considered pathognomonic. Occasionally, erythematous patches which sometimes may ulcerate, occur in the skin over the peripheral joints, such as knuckles, knees and ankles. Hyperemia of the skin and tissues around the fingernails may be present. Haserick has emphasized the fact that the erythema on the hand in dermatomyositis, although closely resembling that seen in systemic lupus erythematosus, can be differentiated from the erythema in systemic lupus erythematosus by its characteristic distribution. In dermatomyositis, the erythematous involvement does not extend from the knuckles down along the extensor tendons as it does often in systemic lupus erythematosus.

Scleroderma-like effects and Raynaud's phenomenon, although not typical of dermatomyositis, are associated features which may occur with the more typical physical manifestations. The cuticle may extend over the nail plate, forming a pterygium similar to that seen in other diseases associated with interference of arterial blood flow to the digits.

Arthritis and arthralgias and effusions of the small joints of the fingers and wrists occur in about half the patients with polymyositis and may be the initial manifestations of the disease. Muscular weakness and cutaneous and arthritic features may predate the discovery of a malignant lesion by as much as two years.

SYSTEMIC LUPUS ERYTHEMATOSUS

In the acute disseminated form of systemic lupus erythematosus the cutaneous lesions begin as erythematous patches on the face, involving the classic "butterfly area" covering the cheeks, nose, eyelids, ears and the "V" area of the neck. This dyscollagenosis also demonstrates a high level of photosensitivity and involves the hands,

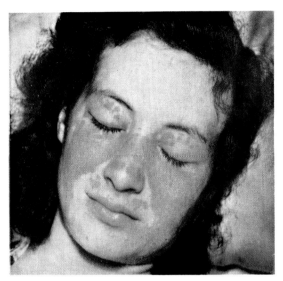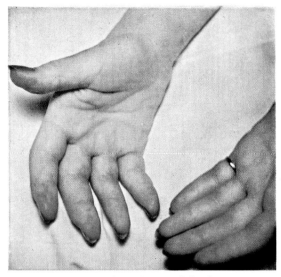

Fig. 39. Systemic lupus erythematosus. Classic "butterfly rash" on the face and erythema of the finger-tips. Raynaud's phenomenon is frequently observed in this and other dyscollagenoses. (Courtesy of Ormsby and Montgomery: Diseases of the Skin, 7th ed. Lea & Febiger.)

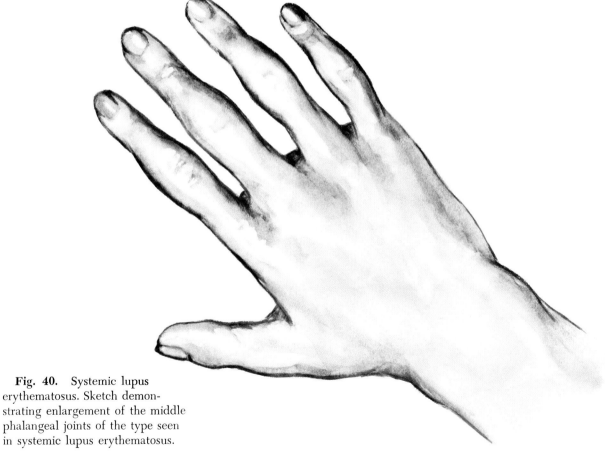

Fig. 40. Systemic lupus erythematosus. Sketch demonstrating enlargement of the middle phalangeal joints of the type seen in systemic lupus erythematosus.

particularly the fingertips. On the hands it may be erythematous, papular or purpuric. The reddening of the dorsum of the hand extends from the cuticle proximally in a linear fashion, over the knuckles and along the extensor tendons. Early in the disease the ends of the fingers may be a bright scarlet, but later become cyanotic. A type of Raynaud's phenomenon occurs fairly frequently in systemic lupus erythematosus.

Arthritic manifestations are observed in the hands of patients with systemic lupus erythematosus, and are similar morphologically and symptomatically to those of rheumatoid arthritis. However, the associated signs of local inflammation are not usually found. In certain instances there may be marked deformity, x-ray changes, and muscle wasting which closely resembles that seen in advanced stages of rheumatoid arthritis. It is not uncommon for the patient with early systemic lupus erythematosus to exhibit joint involvement for many years before symptoms and signs of disease appear in other parts of the body.

THE CARPAL-TUNNEL SYNDROME

The carpal-tunnel syndrome is due to compression of the median nerve, or perhaps stems from ischemic changes in the carpal tunnel at the wrist. It is frequently due to rheumatoid arthritis, or tenosynovitis at the wrist. Other less common causes are amyloid disease, gout, plasmacytoma and fractures, and it has occurred following a bee sting. An association with the endocrine system is suggested by the frequency with which this condition is noted in pregnancy, the menopause, acromegaly and myxedema.

Characteristic symptoms include nocturnal acroparesthesias which may waken the patient. This type of pain, described as a tingling, burning or bursting sensation in the area of the hand supplied by the median nerve, is probably due to peripheral vasodilatation that occurs during sleep. It never involves the little finger and only rarely the thumb. The patient may offer the information that the symptoms are relieved by putting the hands outside the bedclothing, or by immersing them in cold water.

As the condition progresses the pain and neurologic effects become irreversible. On examination, a loss of sensation in the area of the hand supplied by the median nerve can be detected, and wasting of muscles in the thenar group occurs.

The syndrome is encountered five times more often in women than in men, and most frequently in the menopausal age group. Diagnosis is suggested by the classic history of nocturnal pain relieved by cooling the hand, and by the wrist flexion test. In this pro-

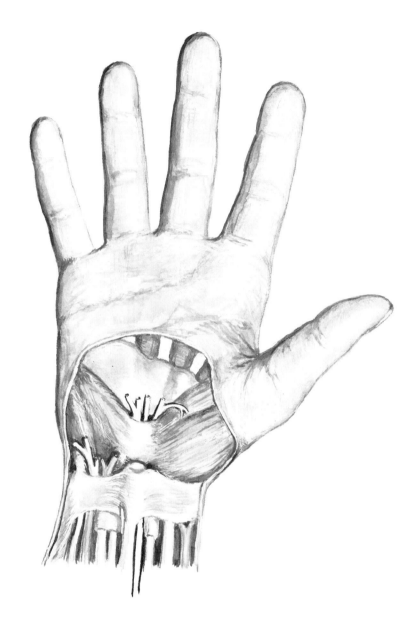

Fig. 41. Anatomy of the carpal tunnel, showing the median nerve in its anatomic relationship within the carpal tunnel.

Fig. 42. Test for the carpal tunnel syndrome. By having the patient with the carpal tunnel syndrome perform this maneuver, pain is reproduced along the distribution of the median nerve owing to exaggerating this nerve's compression in the carpal tunnel.

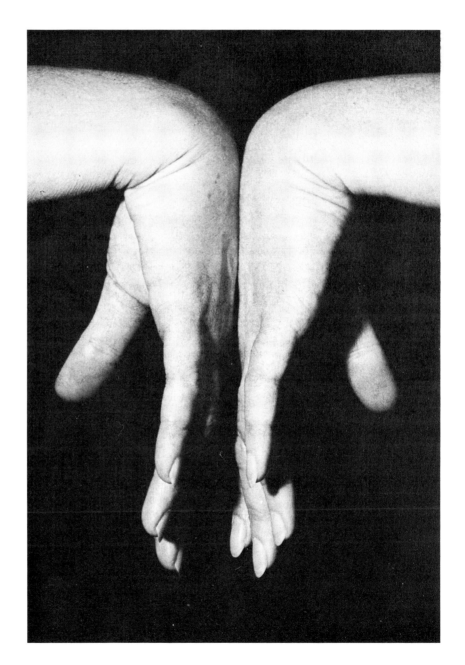

Fig. 43A. Boeck's sarcoid. Middle phalangeal arthropathy resembling the distribution seen in rheumatoid arthritis.

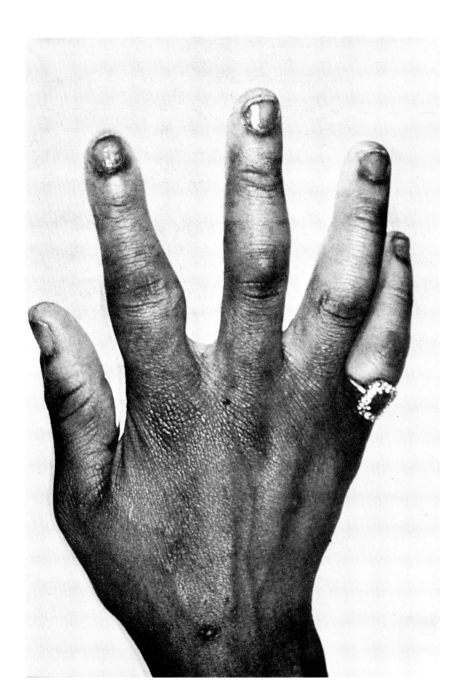

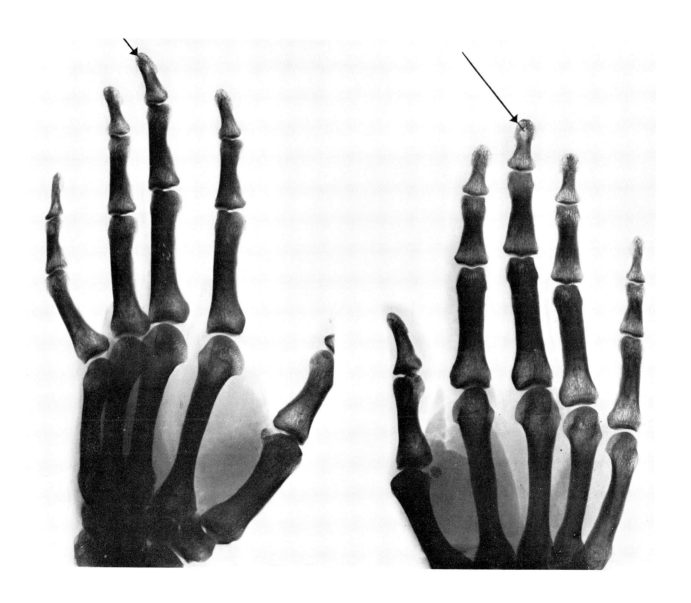

Fig. 43B.   Roentgenogram of hand in Boeck's sarcoid showing punched-out rarefaction in the distal phalanx.

vocative test the dorsums of each hand are forcefully pressed together with the fingers pointing downward. By exaggerating the compression of the median nerve the typic pain pattern is reproduced. A similar compressing maneuver may be produced by inflation of a blood pressure cuff above the wrist of the patient for 30 to 60 seconds, by which the characteristic pain is duplicated in the area of median nerve distribution.

Included in the differential diagnosis are costoclavicular compression, cervical rib and the superior thoracic outlet syndrome (scalenus anticus, etc.).

SARCOIDOSIS

According to reports in the medical literature, about half the patients with systemic sarcoidosis manifest some form of cutaneous disturbance, and slightly less than 20 per cent have roentgen-ray changes in the bones of the hands and feet. These bony changes are due to rarefaction and trabeculation of the medullary part of the phalanges and the metacarpals, or to punched out areas in the small bones of the feet and hands. However, in three large metropolitan hospitals we could find only one roentgenogram in the teaching files to illustrate classic osseous changes of sarcoidosis. We suspect the quoted figure of incidence is inordinately high, at least in Philadelphia.

Fibrous nodules are sometimes seen at the interphalangeal joints and the deformity in the fingers may resemble the type usually seen in rheumatoid arthritis. The associated periarticular swelling produces stiffness and tightness so that mobility is impaired in these joints.

Paronychia are frequent in the early stages of sarcoidosis. A curious type of unidigital clubbing, in which the distal phalanx may be enlarged and flattened dorsoventrally, is sometimes present.

REITER'S SYNDROME

Reiter's syndrome refers to a triad of arthritis, nonspecific urethritis and purulent conjunctivitis. It was first described as a combined clinical entity in 1818 and was named subsequently for Reiter, who grouped the features in a diagnostic package almost one hundred years later.

Involvement of the weight-bearing joints is most commonly encountered, but in many instances the wrist and fingers may be affected. The arthritic disturbance is usually unilateral, seldom bi-

Fig. 44. Reiter's syndrome. Nail changes and signs of inflammation in the tissues surrounding the nails constitute part of the mucocutaneous lesions of Reiter's syndrome. (Courtesy of R. M. Poske, M.D., Annals of Internal Medicine. Montgomery, Poske, Barton, Foxworthy & Baker.)

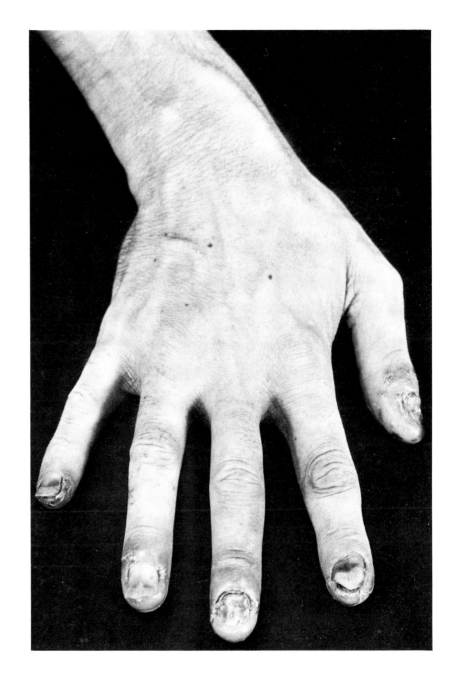

lateral or symmetric. This distribution of arthropathy is suggestive of Reiter's syndrome, particularly when either or both of the other members of the triad are present. Weight loss, balanitis, mild transient diarrhea and an accelerated erythrocyte sedimentation rate are other associated clinical features. Mucocutaneous lesions are found with sufficient frequency to permit their inclusion in what has been more recently regarded as a *tetrad* of Reiter's syndrome.

Hyperkeratosis and nail changes occur in about 30 per cent of patients with this syndrome. Toenails and fingernails are affected in most patients, with loss of one or more nails. Subungual abscesses and keratoses on the fingers and toes are common. The nails become discolored and yellow, and dry debris collects beneath the distal half. As keratin builds up, the nail is elevated, turns dark brown or is blackened and eventually is shed. The skin adjacent to the nail is usually involved.

The clinical features in this syndrome are to be differentiated from those of psoriasis, which Reiter's syndrome closely resembles. Absence of urethral discharge and conjunctivitis in psoriasis is an outstanding point of differentiation. Seasonal relapse and remissions do not occur in Reiter's syndrome.

PACHYDERMOPERIOSTOSIS (the Syndrome of Touraine, Solente and Golé)

Pachydermoperiostosis is a curious and rare disorder in which a number of skin and connective tissue defects are noted. The abnormal physical features include a fusiform cortical thickening of the middle and proximal phalanges bilaterally; clubbed, oversized fingers; "water-glassed" nails and deep sagittal ridging of the scalp. The transverse creases of the forehead are exaggerated, producing deep disfiguring furrows. The skin of the palm, especially on the hypothenar pad, demonstrates a strange rippled arrangement that looks somewhat like finely ridged, water-ribbed sand.

HERITABLE DISORDERS OF CONNECTIVE TISSUE

Many of us in clinical medicine have acquired habits which we indulge by sorting through pathologic material in search for common biologic denominators. The heritable diseases offer a fascinating field for such speculative exercises. Particularly provocative are those genetic misadventures which involve primarily the connective tissues. A partial list includes the Marfan syndrome, Ehlers-Danlos syndrome, pseudoxanthoma elasticum, osteogenesis imperfecta and epidermolysis bullosa. Although it is generally conceded to belong

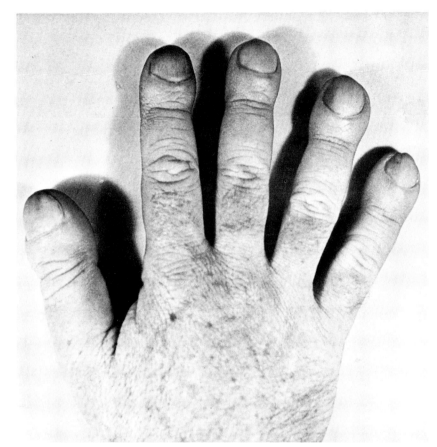

Fig. 45. Clubbed fingers due to Pachydermoperiostosis.

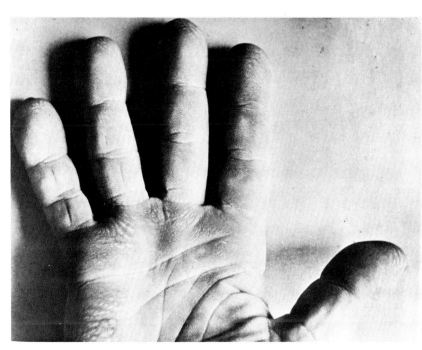

Fig. 46. Pachydermoperiostosis. Note clubbing of the fingers, thickness of the digits, and ridging of the skin of the palm. In this rare syndrome, thickening of the skin exaggerates the creases in the forehead, and deep, coarse, sagittal furrows appear in the scalp.

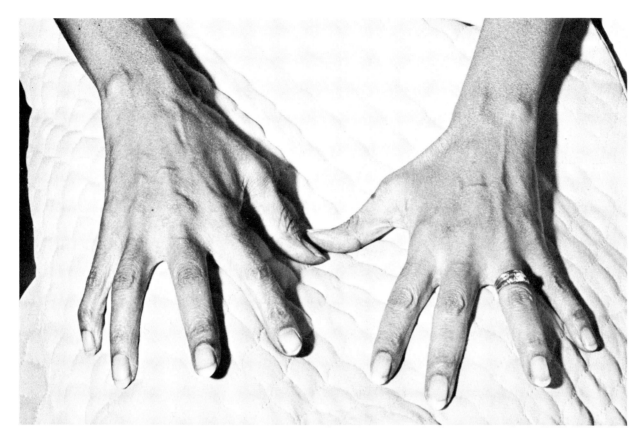

Fig. 47.   Sickle cell disease. Slender, supple, delicate hands conform to the general bodily asthenic **habitus** often present in the individual with sickle cell disease.

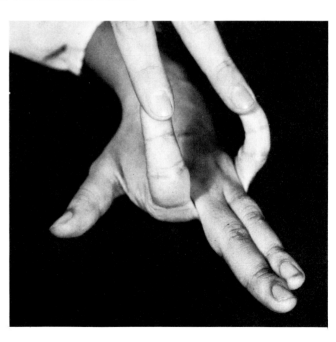

Fig. 48.   Ehlers-Danlos syndrome. Excessive mobility and flexibility of the joints characteristic of the syndrome is demonstrated in this photograph. Fragile, stretchable, rubbery skin and the frequent association with hiatal hernia and intestinal diverticula are features related to the basic defect in collagen structure. (Courtesy of R. M. Goodman, M.D., Johns Hopkins Hospital.)

CONNECTIVE TISSUE

with the blood dyscrasias, there are facets of sickle cell disease which support the inclination to add it categorically to these diseases.

Each of these syndromes is a genetically conditioned disorder which has distinguishing physical effects in the general bodily habitus, and especially in the connective tissue of the skin, extremities and eyes, and in the vascular structures. An outstanding characteristic in the hands of these patients is an exceptional flexibility, or loose-jointed appearance. The fingers are slender and long, the palms narrow, and the movements of the hands are usually serpentine and gracile.

Both *sickle cell disease* and *Marfan's syndrome* have arachnodactyly and long spidery extremities in common. In Marfan's syndrome the focus of attention is centered on the cardiovascular weaknesses, the linear alignment of the frame, and ligamentous laxity. However, in the patient with sickle cell disease, the clinical picture is dominated by the sickling phenomenon of the erythrocytes, and the dramatic, painful "hemolytic crises." When viewed through the other end of the glass, the hematologic defect becomes a mere integer in a combination of systemic involvements by a basic genetic mishap. Other somatic deviations, such as the slender build and osseous changes and the "tower skull" are frequently encountered in sicklers.

In the *Ehlers-Danlos syndrome* there is a subtle similarity to other members of this group, represented by an exceptional degree of extensibility in the fingers which makes it possible to bend back the digits into incredibly unnatural positions. The "India rubber man" is an example of an individual having this syndrome; such a person can usually bend his fingers back until his fingernails touch the face of his wrist watch. Other abnormalities are noted in the heart and blood vessels, and in the dentition. A bleeding tendency is manifest in these patients, who are susceptible to episodes of gastrointestinal hemorrhage.

Epidermolysis bullosa is another connective tissue disorder in which the elastin component is defective. The physical findings are reshuffled and redistributed in an apparently disconnected new combination, but with recognizable modalities familiar to the group. These include a clawed hand, deformed by acquired webbing, and wedged distal phalanges, extensive dental deterioration and stenotic lesions in the esophagus. The fingernails undergo extreme degrees of atrophy and shortening. Frequently the distorted nail plates are shed, leaving deformed, stubby fingertips.

We have had the opportunity to observe a Negress with an interesting combination of heritable diseases—electrophoretically proved sickle cell disease and *pseudoxanthoma elasticum*. This patient had

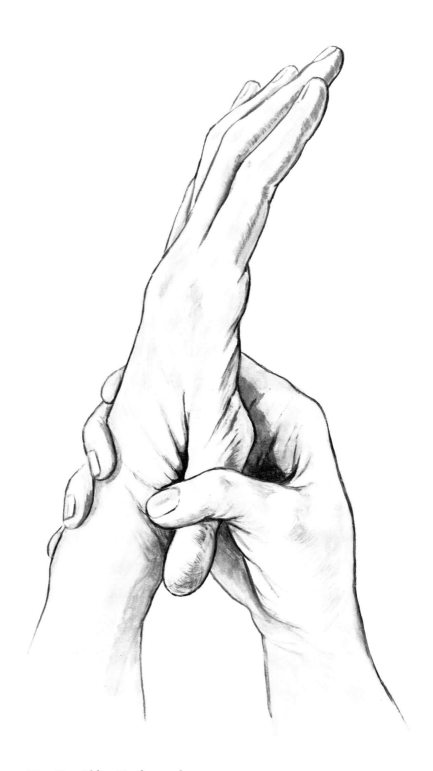

Fig. 49.   Ehlers-Danlos syndrome.

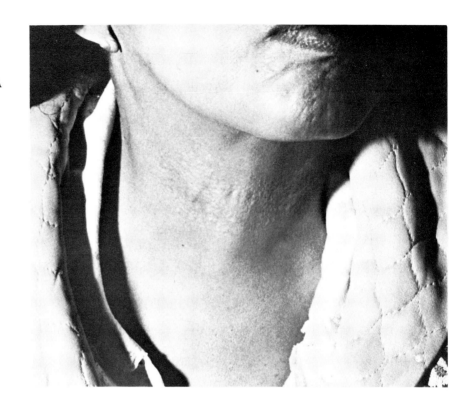

A

B

Fig. 50. Pseudoxanthoma elasticum. A, Crinkly, xanthoma-like lesion on the neck. B, Hands of the same patient; slender, hyperextensible, tapered fingers. Patient also has sickle cell disease.

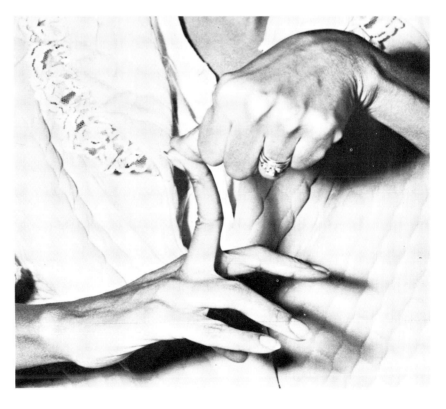

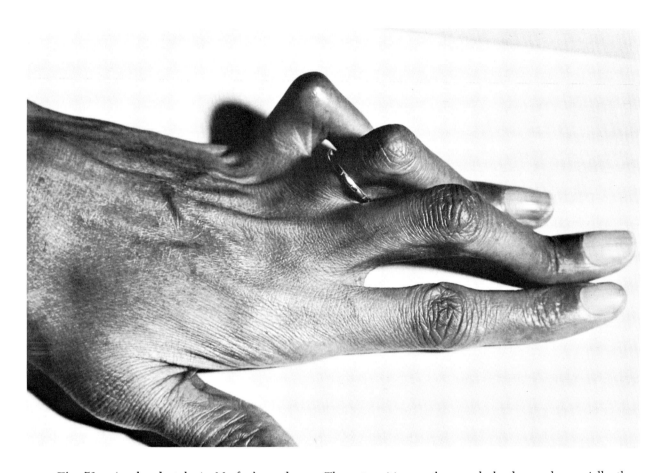

Fig. 51. Arachnodactyly in Marfan's syndrome. The extremities are long and slender, and especially the digits which are called spider fingers. Classically associated with a variety of other skeletal deformities and laxity in the supporting tissues of the cardiovascular system and other areas in the body.

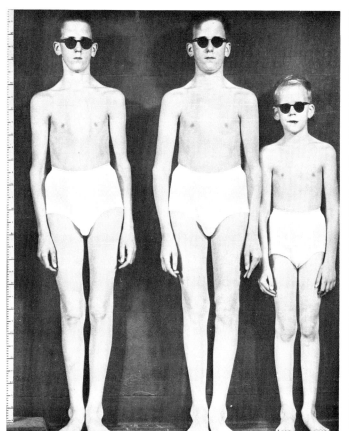
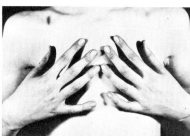
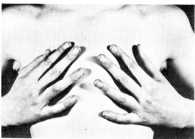
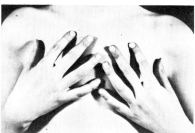

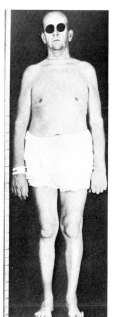
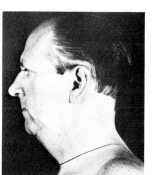
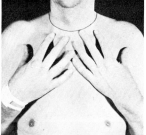

Figs. 52 & 53. Marfan's syndrome. Father and three sons, including twins, all of whom have the bodily configuration of Marfan's syndrome, including arachnodactyly. Note the striking similarity in the form of the hands. (Courtesy of Thomas Killip, III, M.D., Annals of Internal Medicine.)

slender, delicate hands rather than classic arachnodactyly, and an increased extensibility in her fingers more akin to the elastic tissue peculiarities of the Ehlers-Danlos syndrome.

The formes frustes of these diseases may be more prevalent than is realized, and when cross-mixtures occur, as indeed they might, the clinician is faced with a tacky problem in differential diagnosis. The seeker of common denominators and associations in diseases needs no reminder that genetic abnormalities frequently occur in multiples, and the detection of one should stimulate a search for others.

MARFAN'S SYNDROME

The tall, angular, "eccentric dancer," and some of the loose, lean, long men who exploit their exceptional anatomies on basketball courts, are reminiscent of a clinical entity of some importance that goes by the eponym of Marfan's syndrome. Identification is usually possible on simple inspection, and is of importance rather for its prognostic potential than for any therapeutic consideration. A high percentage (approximately 90 per cent) of such people demonstrate several types of cardiovascular catastrophe, many of whom succumb early in life from these effects.

The etiologic basis is unknown, but the pathologic features are nicely catalogued in a widespread involvement of connective tissue throughout the body. These clinical features eventuate apparently from a genetic defect in the mesoderm. Generalized laxity of various ligaments and supportive structures allows for subluxation of the ocular lenses and instability of joints, augmented by a concomitant, defective development of subcutaneous and muscular tissues.

Associated defects in osseous structures account for several of the other features in this curious syndrome, such as occur in the skull, palate, thorax, spine and in the extremities. Angular, elongated, slender limbs and digits contribute to the characteristic spidery form in the fingers which are exceptionally gracile and hyperextensible (arachnodactyly). The hand and arm spans are remarkably long and delicate. When these stigmata are noted in an unusually tall individual, the existence of a mesodermal developmental disorder such as Marfan's syndrome is to be considered. Varying degrees of involvement, and the presence of but a few parts of the syndrome occur more frequently than one would suppose so that the "partial Marfan's" picture is a clinical entity commonly overlooked. Spider fingers (arachnodactylia) are present in some patients suffering from sickle cell disease, but differentiation from Marfan's syndrome poses no great problem. Hyperhemolysis and abdominal crises are not observed in Marfan's syndrome.

OSTEOGENESIS IMPERFECTA

Osteogenesis imperfecta or fragilitas ossium is another heritable disorder with multiple mesenchymal defects which demonstrates a characteristic slender, delicate configuration in the hand. In this disease, which resembles osteoporosis, multiple fractures occur in various bones throughout the body, usually from minimal traumas. For some unknown reason the fragility of osseous structures seems to lessen after adolescence.

Major clinical characteristics of osteogenesis imperfecta are the blue sclerae, "box-head" deformity, multiple fractures and the delicate hand seen in other members of this disease group.

STENOSING TENOSYNOVITIS (deQuervain's Syndrome)

This condition is caused by constriction of a tendon by its retaining fibrous ligament. The constriction produces an irritation and, ultimately, an inflammatory process which interferes with the free gliding movement of the tendon in its sheath. It is, apparently, related to an endocrine disorder and to a generalized alteration of collagen. This condition is most commonly found in people who perform manual work and involves the right hand more often than the left. Individuals in their middle forties are most often affected. Constriction produces pain in the affected tendon, which is swollen, and causes a snapping sensation in the area of involvement. Pain may be sufficiently severe to be disabling.

The most common sites of involvement are (1) in the sheaths which enclose the tendons of the abductor pollicis longus and extensor pollicis brevis; (2) the sheaths of the flexor sublimis and profundus tendons of the middle two fingers; (3) the sheath of the flexor pollicis longus at the metacarpophalangeal joints.

A stenosing tenosynovitis of the flexor tendons of the fingers may cause pain and snapping at the metacarpophalangeal joint and produce the so-called "trigger finger" deformity. The ring and middle fingers are most frequently involved. There is often tenderness at the neck of the metacarpal bones and a firm swelling is palpable at the same area. Ganglia sometimes form on the fibrous sheaths in association with stenosing tenosynovitis of the fingers.

The carpal tunnel syndrome is similar to a stenosing tenosynovitis. The median nerve which is encroached upon in the canal with the long flexor tendons produces symptoms earlier, before a stenosing effect has had time to develop.

3

diseases of the NERVOUS SYSTEM

The distribution of nerves in the upper extremity is relatively uncomplicated, and zoning of sensory and motor control through the median, ulnar and radial nerves follows a fairly regular anatomic pattern. These three major nerve trunks spring from the cervical plexus, and carry both sensory and motor components. Interruption of the nerve pathways to the hand may be caused by trauma, infection, or by degenerative process, or encroachment by tumor, producing definitive physical signs. Atrophy or paresis results from interference with the neural circuit at any level from the cerebral cortex to the peripheral branches, and each level produces characteristic physical changes.

Following peripheral nerve injury, sudomotor activity is impaired in a segmental fashion, a clinically useful fact in both diagnosis and prognosis. The area of anhidrosis corresponds closely to the zone of functional loss or anesthesia. Objective measurement of sweat gland function is possible by the use of simple tests for detection of chloride excretion. The palm of the injured hand is pressed against a piece of specially prepared, silver-impregnated filter paper. Chloride from the normally innervated sweat glands forms a precipitate quickly, and thus allows for a comparison with the uninjured hand. Healing and subsequent return of sudomotor activity can be recorded and preserved for medicolegal or prognostic purposes. With careful observation the same phenomenon may be discernible with the unaided eye.

Occasionally a segmental, congenital absence of sweat glands in a

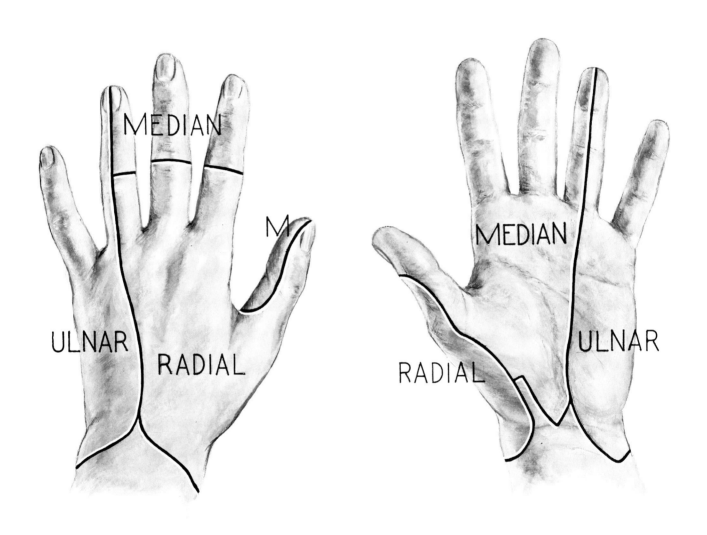

Fig. 54. Nerve distribution in the hand.

part of the palm may be noted, but has no clinical importance. The skin in the anhidrotic area has a finely crinkled and somewhat roughened appearance.

In this chapter are included descriptions of various types of tremor, the major palsies which involve the hand, and several systemic neurologic, demyelinating or degenerative diseases of the central and peripheral nerves.

TREMOR

Several types of tremor which may affect various parts of the body, such as the chin, head, the tongue or extremities, are encountered in clinical medicine. Differentiation of the several kinds of tremor may be possible on bedside examination, and allow the examiner to arrive at a correct diagnosis. Certain tremors are sufficiently characteristic to be disease-specific, while others are merely associated accompaniments of a generalized neuromuscular disorder.

In a general way, tremor might be considered as a resultant of altered muscular tonus, an extrapyramidal tract sign not increased on intention and usually exaggerated by nervous excitation.

Tremors have been classified arbitrarily according to their amplitude, regularity, location and relationship to voluntary movements or effort. An *action* tremor, for example, is one which occurs when the limbs are actively maintained in a particular position. It is generally more rapid, less regular, and finer in amplitude than are static tremors. An *intention* tremor, in contrast, occurs during purposeful, wilful movements and is generally coarse and jerky. This variety of tremor disappears during repose.

Most often an irregular tremor of the hand has no more useful diagnostic significance than to act as an indicator of a situational nervousness in a tense individual faced with the stressful experience of submitting to the physical examination itself. This type of patient may display other telltale effects of anxiety, and especially by his hands, which are frequently restless, cool and wet with perspiration during the examination. Usually, by the time the interview has been completed the tremor of the hand has disappeared in those instances when it was caused by simple anxiety.

Tremor may be observed in several medically important systemic conditions such as hyperthyroidism, neurocirculatory asthenia, paralysis agitans, multiple sclerosis, cerebral or cerebellar disorders, hepatolenticular degeneration, hypoglycemia, occupational neuroses and in certain toxic states.

FAMILIAL TREMOR

A familial type of tremor is not uncommon, and has no especial disease significance, except as a potential detriment to fine manual work under certain stressful circumstances. A heritable trait, it seems to be transmitted as a mendelian dominant which is, for the most part, associated with the male sex. Familial tremor may occur early in life, but usually begins in the third decade. It is rapid and regular and fine in character. It is not affected by position or intention, although it becomes exaggerated when the individual is aware of being watched. The intake of food has no effect on its presence, although a salutary influence is apparent after the use of social doses of alcohol.

HYPERTHYROIDISM

The tremor in hyperthyroidism consists of a fine trembling of the hands and rarely affects other parts of the body. Its occurrence in the characteristically warm, satiny-skinned hand is diagnostically helpful (see *Hyperthyroidism*).

NEUROCIRCULATORY ASTHENIA

Often the anxiety produced by a clinical examination, or the fears related to the consequences of his illness, are sufficiently provocative to set the neurasthenic's hands into motion. Usually the tremor is coarse and irregular, both in amplitude and in time of manifestation. The hands are invariably cold and wet, and in almost constant motion during the examination. Restless, intertwining, writhing movements are punctuated by frequent neurotic picking, scratching, stroking and probing gestures to the face, hair and clothing. Punctilious straightening of attire and office furnishings, the wringing of the handkerchief and the nervous examination of the fingernails and cuticle demonstrated by the neurasthenic individual offer dynamic testimony of the patient's emotional reserves, and contrast sharply with the calm, quiet demeanor of the person whose hands lie still.

PARALYSIS AGITANS

The parkinsonian tremor is of the static variety and affects one or both hands when they are at repose. It ceases momentarily upon the execution of a conscious purposeful movement. The hand generally "lacks expression," owing to the presence of rigidity which is an outstanding characteristic of Parkinson's disease. One might consider this tremor to be an example of interrupted rigidity. The tremor of the extremity in parkinsonism is coarse and of a large amplitude, sometimes with an excursion of many inches. Often it vanishes miraculously when the individual performs a manual act, such as drinking from a cup, so that he seldom has serious difficulty eating or drinking. The "pill-rolling palsy" describes itself, and is one of the cardinal neuromuscular features of paralysis agitans.

The parkinsonian tremor may be encountered in persons with severe head injury, carbon monoxide poisoning, manganese toxicity, vascular accident and cerebral degeneration due to arteriosclerosis.

ATHETOSIS

In this dynamic neuromuscular sign, the hands and fingers are contorted through a series of endless sinuous, writhing, purposeless movements, with alternate flexion and extension of the digits. The term "athetosis" is derived from the Greek word which means "unfixed" or "changeable." Athetosis occurs in a variety of disease states and can be classified according to three general types: double, unilateral and bilateral athetosis.

Double athetosis is a term applied to an infantile type which is thought to be a developmental anomaly, or related possibly to certain toxic phenomena, birth trauma, or to asphyxic injury occurring at birth.

Athetoid movements are not apparent immediately after birth. These abnormal gyrations are not usually perceptible until the age is reached when the uncertain, infantile manual functions normally become more dexterous. By about the eighth or ninth month of life the healthy infant begins to show definite signs of developing some crude control of hand movement and dexterity. At this stage of development the fingers of the athetoid child are seen to behave in an abnormal way, demonstrated by slow twisting, vermicular movements and grotesque posturing of the hands.

Unilateral or bilateral athetosis is usually secondary to a cerebral lesion, such as hemorrhage. Lateralization corresponds to the location of the central disorder. Athetosis which is sequela to hemiplegia is rather rare in adults, and is much more commonly related to cerebrovascular accidents in children. When it occurs in childhood it usually persists throughout life.

The wild contortions of the athetotic hand may traumatize seriously the emotional system of the afflicted individual, who often attempts to control the defect by sitting on his hands. Many patients with tremor of the hands from any cause will assume the same attitude, or place their hands in their pockets to hide their disability.

SYDENHAM'S CHOREA

The movements of Sydenham's chorea, an infection of the brain related, in many instances, to acute tonsillitis, acute rheumatic fever or endocarditis, are described by Neison as "involuntary, unexpected, sudden, nonrhythmic, irregular, purposeless, forced movements of wide excursion, which affect the proximal portion of the limbs more than the distal, in contrast to the findings of athetosis."

HUNTINGTON'S CHOREA

Huntington's chorea, which disturbs the gait and the fine movements of the hands, is an hereditary disease due to degeneration of ganglionic cells in the corpus striatum and cortex, with reduction of the volume of white matter. The early symptoms begin in adult life, usually with either forced movements or with dementia, later with ataxia and choreiform movements in the hands. The hands and arms are twisted through the most grotesque movements, and the fingers, unlike those of the patient with Sydenham's chorea, are involved in the process rather than the proximal portions of the limbs.

HYPOGLYCEMIA

When the blood glucose concentration reaches a critical low level an irregular fine tremor of the hand is generally perceptible. Commonly observed as a result of hyperinsulinism, from either exogenous or endogenous sources, it also occurs occasionally in otherwise normal people who display only mild symptoms of functional hypoglycemia. Understandably, it appears most often in the late morning before luncheon, or in the late afternoon before dinner. It is worsened after vigorous exercise or excessive usage of tobacco. This type of tremor is relieved dramatically by the ingestion of adequate amounts of carbohydrate or raw sugars.

TREMOR IN HEPATIC DISEASE

Certain metabolic abnormalities of cerebral function are related to hepatic disease. Recent investigations have more accurately delineated several different hepatic enzyme deficits as first causes for altered biochemical liver-brain relationships. Examples of hepatic encephalopathic syndromes which seem to affect primarily the function of the basal ganglia are hepatic coma, Wilson's hepatolenticular degeneration, and the postinfectious hepatitic state. In each of these conditions a characteristic tremor of the hand resembling that seen in parkinsonism is present.

Wilson's Disease (Hepatolenticular Degeneration)

Tremor is a cardinal symptom in Wilson's disease. Frequently the first sign to appear, it is always a prominent clinical feature. Initially the tremor is fine in character, has a limited range, and is regular at about four to eight oscillations per second. Voluntary movement and physical or mental exertion accentuate it. As the disease progresses further along in its course, tremor becomes more extensive and eventually involves the entire body.

Beginning at the same time as the tremor appears, or shortly thereafter, rigidity develops and finally produces contracture deformities in the extremities. Voluntary movements cause the tremor to simulate that of paralysis agitans or chorea. (See also discussion of Wilson's disease on page 117.)

Hepatic Coma

The quick, flapping tremor of impending hepatic coma is similar to the tremor noted in parkinsonism except it is not associated with rigidity. It is amplified by having the patient hold his arms out at his side, which causes the hands and upper extremities to flap in a manner suggesting a wing-beating motion. Such a tremor is an ominous sign, one which is reliable as an indicator of early decompensation of hepatic function.

Posthepatitic Tremor

A parkinsonian type of tremor has been described as a late and uncommon sequela of infectious hepatitis (viral). It is not usually associated with rigidity or sialorrhea.

MULTIPLE SCLEROSIS

In multiple sclerosis the tremor is of the intention type and is almost always present to some degree. It involves the head and trunk as well as the limbs. When the patient with multiple sclerosis is

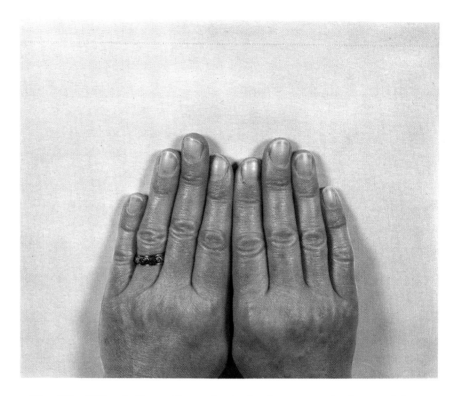

Fig. 55. Wilson's disease (hepatolenticular degeneration). Abnormal depositions of copper are found in the brain, liver and cornea in Wilson's disease. Deposits of copper may occur in the nail moons, as shown in these hands, producing an azure coloration. (Courtesy of Alexander G. Bearn, M.D.—Bearn and McKusick: J.A.M.A. 166:904.)

asked to touch his nose with his fingertip he may execute the move properly, but the tremor is accentuated when the finger arrives at its goal. The tremor is absent in bed or at rest.

When this type of "action tremor" is found in conjunction with a scanning speech and nystagmus the diagnosis of multiple sclerosis must be considered.

FRONTAL LOBE LESIONS

A fine tremor of the contralateral hand is encountered in frontal lobe lesions. It is made worse when the hand is used, and participates in the so-called "frontal ataxia" seen in patients with disease of that area.

GENERAL PARALYSIS OF THE INSANE AND LESIONS OF THE RED NUCLEUS

In general paralysis of the insane there is a rhythmic tremor of the outstretched hand. Lesions of the red nucleus are also likely to produce a fine tremor of the hands, best seen when the hands are held outstretched and the fingers spread. The tremor involves the contralateral hand and will cease when the hand is at rest; it is usually associated with an ipsilateral palsy of the third cranial nerve.

CEREBELLAR TREMORS

Cerebellar tremors are of the intention type, and are ipsilateral, coarse, irregular oscillations, which are accentuated by the finger-nose test. The tremor is amplified as the finger approaches its target.

OTHER TREMORS

Other causes of tremor in the hand are *exposure to cold, fatigue,* and exogenous *intoxications* from alcohol, heavy metals or barbiturates. *Narcotic* addicts exhibit coarse tremors of the hand as part of the withdrawal symptomatology.

THE THUMB IN DIAGNOSTIC SCREENING OF PARALYSIS

The development of a thumb capable of a rotary motion, with ability to oppose with each of the other fingers, has contributed more to man's rise above the remainder of the animal kingdom than

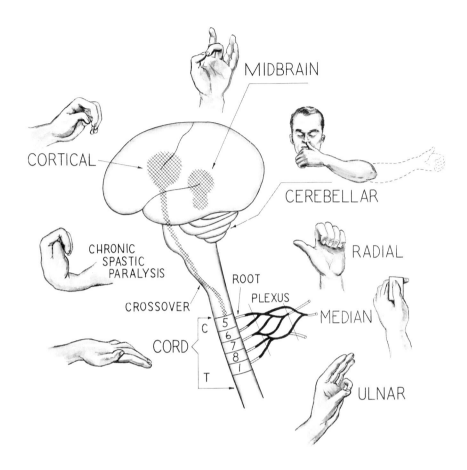

Fig. 56. Thumb signs and screening tests for localization of lesions at various levels in the nervous system.

1. CORTICAL LESIONS. In oncoming cortical spastic paralysis the thumb is flexed and drawn into the palm. In chronic spastic paralysis the thumb is held firmly by the flexed fingers; the wrist is acutely flexed.

2. MIDBRAIN LESIONS. The patient with involvement of the extrapyramidal system and other deep central brain disorders usually is unable to touch repeatedly and rapidly the tip of the thumb to the top of the middle finger.

3. CEREBELLAR THUMB. Test for cerebellar dysmetria (see text); this procedure will also aid in the detection of certain types of tremor.

4. CORD THUMB. Pathologic conditions affecting the spinal cord, or the roots of the sixth, seventh and eighth cervical nerves, cause atrophy of the intrinsic muscles of the hand. The hand appears flattened and the tip of the thumb can be positioned completely behind the knuckle of the index finger.

5. TEST FOR RADIAL NERVE PARALYSIS. Sketch showing thumb-cocked position which cannot be assumed by patient with radial nerve paralysis.

6. ULNAR THUMB. In paralysis of ulnar nerve the thumb cannot touch the tip of the little finger across the palm.

7. MEDIAN THUMB. The patient with paralysis of the median nerve cannot pinch the pad of the thumb against the index finger or hold a card in this manner against resistance. In a lesion of the plexus all three of the peripheral nerves may be involved and the physical findings are due to a combination of radial, ulnar and median nerve interference.

NERVOUS SYSTEM   **72**

has any other physiologic or anatomic advancement. Because of the mechanical potential of his thumb, man has been able to achieve a dexterity for skills and arts of incredible fineness and range. By far the most functionally important of the digits, the thumb is also the strongest and most maneuverable, partly because of its location in a plane at right angles to the metacarpals, and its separation from the fingers and palm. The thumb maintains a larger cortical representation in the motor area of the cortex than does any of the other digits.

Temple Fay has formulated a bedside method for rapid screening of neurologic lesions by observation of the mechanics of the patient's thumb; his schema has useful clinical application in the localization of disease in the brain, cord, root, plexus, or in the peripheral nerves. Emphasis is placed on the presence of an abnormal thumb position combined with a Hoffmann's sign as an omen of serious central nervous system involvement.

THUMB TESTS

The following thumb tests have been used as a quick screening guide to the probable location of the causative lesion when paralysis of the upper extremity and hand is encountered. They aid in separating and roughly categorizing those patients whose findings merit more detailed neurologic testing and study.

Cortical Thumb

When the thumb is flexed at the tip, or is tucked into the palm, an oncoming, existing or subsiding phase of cortical spastic paralysis is suggested.

In the spastic paralysis of children the thumb is pointed downward and is usually carried out and away from the body. Adult spastics are inclined to flex the thumb at the wrist, which is usually drawn by flexion toward the chest.

Midbrain Thumb

Defects in function of the deep structures of the brain, such as occur in inflammatory processes, focal lesions of the basal ganglions, and in paralysis agitans, produce a motor weakness whereby the individual cannot rapidly and repeatedly touch the tip of the thumb to the tip of the index or middle finger. Thumb movements are stiff and delayed. In true motor paralysis, movements or portions of movements are weak, uncertain or absent. Free swinging of the arms and coordinated action of the hand in walking are absent. An example of such an effect follows involvement of the basal ganglion by inflammation or degenerative changes. Other characteristic effects include rigidity, dystonia, and parkinsonian syndrome.

Cerebellar Thumb

A simple test of cerebellar disorders is performed by having the patient touch the tip of his thumb to his nose with his eyes closed. The intention tremor of multiple sclerosis is readily observed, or perhaps a cerebellar vestibular ataxia can be identified by the presence of associated dysmetria. Hyperthyroid tremors are persistent, whereas malingerers generally exaggerate the defect. The fine tremor of midbrain lesions disappear with this maneuver. If the individual misses the nose on the first effort, but connects on the second try, particularly if the disturbance affects only one side, an intrinsic cerebellar dysfunction is suggested and further diagnostic survey is necessary.

Cord Thumb

When the spinal cord is involved, as in myelitis, or when a pathologic process includes the nerve roots of the lower cervical cord, such as the sixth, seventh or eighth cervical nerves, atrophy and weakness of the intrinsic muscles of the hand occur. This type of atrophy produces a characteristic appearance that has been called "ape hand" because of the appearance of the thumb which can be placed behind the knuckle of the index finger. When changes follow a segmental pattern they signify lesions or pressure effect involving both motor and sensory modalities, probably localized in the cervical area. When purely motor signs are observed, one should suspect anterior poliomyelitis, amyotrophic lateral sclerosis, or local or focal intrinsic lesions of the cord and roots, such as occur in hematomyelia.

Plexus Thumb

In profound paralysis involving the brachial plexus, a flaccid weakness occurs in which the thumb cannot touch the tips of the other fingers, cannot be held to the side of the index finger, nor can it be cocked backward (radial, median, and ulnar nerves impaired). The three major nerve trunks are affected, so that there is usually a combination of sensory and motor defects.

Ulnar Thumb

Ulnar nerve paralysis makes it impossible for the thumb to oppose with the fifth finger across the palm.

Radial Thumb

In musculospiral nerve paralysis the thumb cannot be cocked backward or held against a resistance. The sensory changes affect the dorsum of the hand around the base of the thumb and adjoining fingers.

Median Thumb

Paralysis of the median nerve makes it impossible for the individual so afflicted to pinch the thumb tightly against the side of the index finger.

MEDIAN NERVE PARALYSIS

The median nerve is well protected by surrounding soft tissues and is less often injured than are the other nerves of the hand and is seldom involved by paralysis alone. Dislocations of the shoulder, injuries at the elbow, or perforating wounds may cause median nerve damage, or the nerve may be compressed in its course through the carpal tunnel by tenosynovitis, tumor or ligamentous hypertrophy.

The hand appears broader than usual owing to flattening of the thenar eminence. The thumb is extended and adducted and drawn back to the same plane as the other fingers. There is inability to pronate the forearm beyond the midposition. The wrist is supinated and can be flexed only toward the ulnar side, and the thumb cannot be opposed to the fingertips. The second phalanges cannot be flexed on the first, and the distal phalanges of the first and second fingers cannot be flexed. The proximal phalanges, however, can still be flexed. Loss of the ability to flex the distal phalanx of the index finger is a pathognomonic sign. Ulnar nerve function can substitute for many of the lost functions of the median nerve except for flexion of the distal phalanx of the index finger and palmar abduction of the thumb.

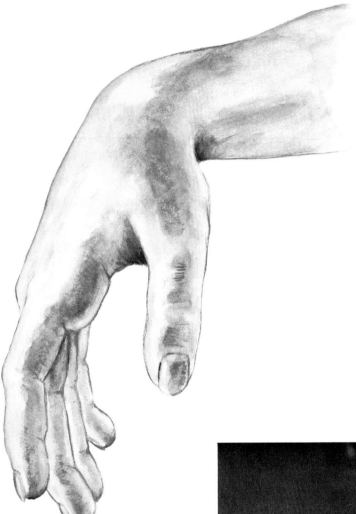

Fig. 57.

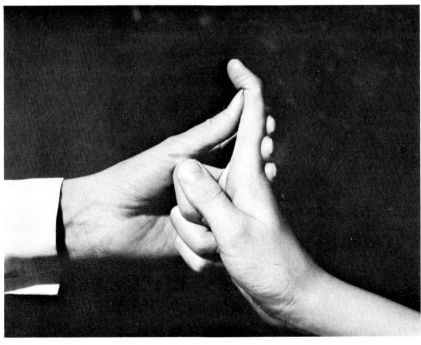

Fig. 57. Wrist drop in radial
nerve paralysis.

Fig. 58

Fig. 58. Test for median
nerve paralysis. The distal phalanx
cannot be flexed on the middle
phalanx in paralysis of the median
nerve.

There is a loss of sensation on the radial side of the palm and the palmar aspect of the thumb, the first two fingers and half of the third finger, the tips of the fingers and the dorsal surfaces of the same three fingers. Wasting of the thenar muscles, which is usually prominent, produces the characteristic "ape hand" or "monkey paw" deformity. Grasping power is lost or lessened in the thumb and index finger.

RADIAL NERVE PARALYSIS

The most frequent of all the peripheral nerve palsies is that which involves the radial nerve. Radial paralysis is incurred most often as a result of a crutch injury or from pressure on the nerve by dislocation of the shoulder, or by fractures about the shoulder joint, or from injuries sustained by the back of a chair. Lead neuropathy will produce a charactertistic radial nerve palsy.

The most charactertistic feature of radial paralysis is wrist drop and an inability to extend the first phalanges of the thumb and fingers. There is usually some impairment of supination and a loss of extension and abduction of the wrist, fingers and thumb. The thumb is flexed and abducted, but some slight power usually remains in extension of the second and third phalanges by means of lumbricales and interossei musculature. The flexors of the fingers are not impaired, but the grip is weakened because the patient cannot complete flexion of the fingers with the wrist flexed owing to weakness of the synergists. Interphalangeal joint flexion is unimpaired. The deformity of radial nerve paralysis can best be demonstrated if the forearm is flexed at the elbow.

Sensation is lost over the posterior and lateral aspect of the forearm, and is lost to a varying extent over the distribution of the radial nerve on the back of the hand. Trophic changes from radial nerve paralysis are minimal.

ULNAR NERVE PARALYSIS

In ulnar nerve paralysis the hand is angled to the radial side (radial tilting), and adduction of the thumb is impossible. The first phalanges cannot be flexed and the others cannot be extended. In longstanding involvement the first phalanges are overtextended and the others are strongly flexed ("benediction hand"). The hypothenar eminence is thinned causing a shallowness in the cup of the palm. There may be anesthesia of the ulnar side of the hand, affecting the two and a half fingers on the dorsum, and one and a half fingers on

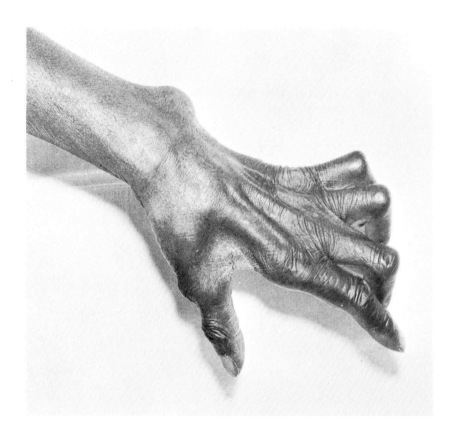

Fig. 59. Ulnar nerve paralysis. "Benediction palsy"—inability to extend fully the fourth and fifth fingers.

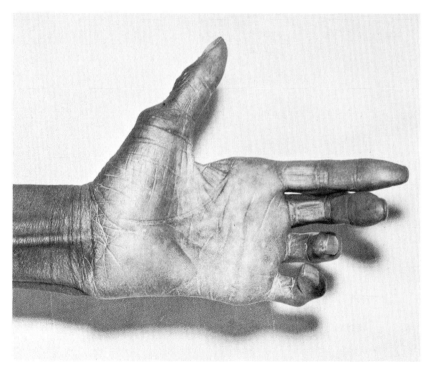

the palmar surfaces. The grasping power is lessened in the fourth and fifth fingers, and the interossei muscles are wasted and unable to abduct or adduct the fingers.

Isolated ulnar nerve paralysis may be caused by certain occupations which allow for pressure on the nerve at the base of the hypothenar eminence, such as occurs in men who use files or vibrating tools. The ulnar nerve is also affected in certain instances in leprosy, chronic lead poisoning, polyarteritis nodosa and hypertrophic polyneuritis.

It may be of diagnostic importance to differentiate ulnar nerve palsies from lesions of the brachial plexus, the eighth cervical nerve root and the cervical cord. Pressure on nerve trunks by a cervical rib can produce weakness or atrophy of muscles of the hand supplied by the ulnar nerve.

Division of the eighth cervical nerve root causes paralysis of all intrinsic muscles of the hand, with a sensory loss only in the medial half of the palm, fifth finger and the entire fourth finger. This is often associated with an ipsilateral Horner's syndrome. Although a traumatic origin is usual, and quite obvious, an extension of a carcinoma from the apex of the lung is an easily overlooked causative mechanism.

The cervical cord may be involved by poliomyelitis, tumor, syringomyelia, hematomyelia, progressive atrophy, or herniation of a cervical intervertebral disk. Tumors of the upper segments of the spinal cord may cause wasting of the small muscles of the hand, and signs of pressure on the long tracts.

AMYOTROPHIC LATERAL SCLEROSIS

Amyotrophic lateral sclerosis is a relentless, incurable, motor nerve disease which usually begins in adult life, and is characterized by progressive muscular atrophy. Involvement may be noted initially in the upper extremity, although the first signs may appear anywhere in the skeletal muscular system. Muscular fasciculations and signs of pyramidal tract involvement are among the early physical findings which progress in a gradual march of muscular wasting and weakness.

Symptomatically, the initial complaints may be related to impairment of the finger movements due to generalized atrophy or weakness of the intrinsic muscles of the hand. The patient may notice slowly increasing clumsiness in writing or in buttoning his clothing, owing to wasting of the interossei muscles and the adductors of the thumbs. There is loss of substance in the thenar and hypothenar muscle masses, which eventually results in a useless, weak hand and painlessly progressive invalidism. Involvement of the respiratory

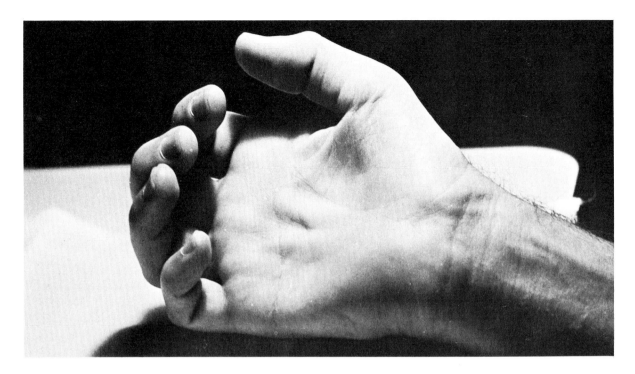

Fig. 60. Amyotrophic lateral sclerosis. Note atrophic effects in the diminished muscle mass in the thenar eminence and in the interossei musculature. Muscle wasting and weakness is painless and progressive in this uniformly fatal disease.

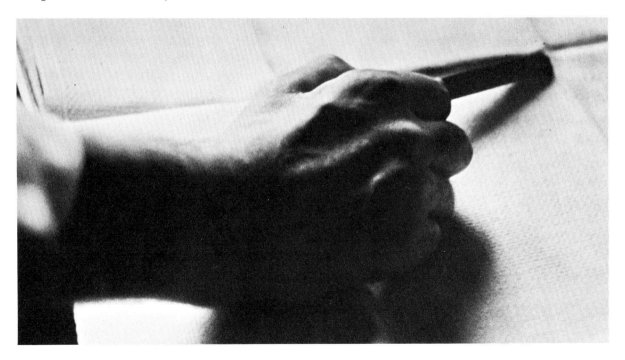

Fig. 61. Amyotrophic lateral sclerosis. This photograph demonstrates atrophy in interossei muscles.

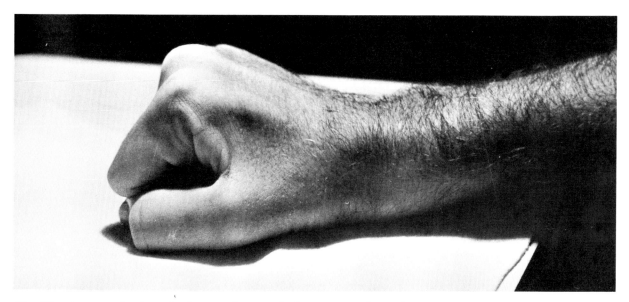

Fig. 62. Amyotrophic lateral sclerosis. Photograph demonstrates diminished mass of the first dorsal interosseous muscle and the adductor pollicis.

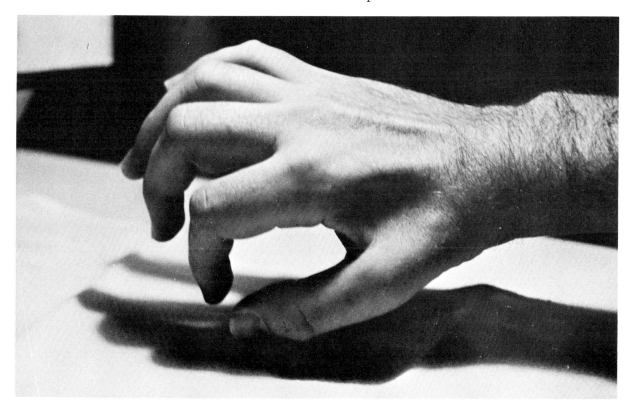

Fig. 63. Amyotrophic lateral sclerosis. Photograph demonstrates diminished mass of the first dorsal interosseous muscle and the adductor pollicis.

center in the bulb and eventual paralysis of ventilation are frequently the terminal mechanisms.

Examination of the hand discloses a generalized painless atrophy of all three main motor nerves, but a complete preservation of sensory nerve function. Fine fasciculations become exaggerated later and are replaced by coarse, jerky movements of the clawed, helpless hand. In later stages the tremor becomes uncontrollable, especially when intense effort is exerted, or when simple muscular maneuvers, such as clenching the fist, are attempted. At first largely unilateral, subsequently the process extends to involve the other hand, and ultimately the lower extremities with the production of foot drop.

Total muscular atrophy in the hand is demonstrated in this disease. Loss of power in the interossei muscles and ulnar nerve makes it difficult or impossible for the patient to hold a pencil in the proper position to write. In early stages the patient will demonstrate interossei weakness by inability to hold a card slotted between the fingers.

Atrophy of adductors of the thumb and the hypothenar group of muscles causes the "ape hand" deformity in which the thumb is held up in a cocked position with its metacarpal lying in the same plane as those of the other digits. The thenar pad is similarly thinned so that the natural hollow of the palm becomes effaced.

CHARCOT-MARIE-TOOTH PERONEAL ATROPHY

Charcot-Marie-Tooth peroneal atrophy is a degenerative disorder of the nervous system which begins usually in childhood and produces atrophy and motor weakness in the small muscles of the feet. Gradual progression to include the other muscles of the leg occurs, and eventually the disease involves the hands. Muscular atrophy usually spares the thighs, so that a disproportion exists between the diameters of the upper and lower leg. The over-all configuration of the limb has been likened to that of an inverted champagne bottle ("ostrich legs"). The deep tendon reflexes are ultimately lost.

Unlike amyotrophic lateral sclerosis, from which it must be differentiated, Charcot-Marie-Tooth atrophy reaches an end point short of fatal bulbar paralysis, permitting a prognosis which is tremendously more favorable. Moreover, the degenerative process begins in the lower leg in this disease and only later involves the hands, whereas, amyotrophic lateral sclerosis usually begins in the hands and, if survival permits, the lower extremities are affected secondarily. In both of these degenerative disorders the atrophic changes in the muscles of the hand are similar, and feature painless "claw hand" deformity due to total myatrophy of the intrinsic musculature.

Fig. 64. Charcot-Marie-Tooth peroneal atrophy. Painless atrophy of the entire hand occurs in many cases of this familial neurologic disease, although the peronei and anterior tibial musculature are usually involved initially. In contrast with amyotrophic lateral sclerosis, which it resembles morphologically in the hands, Charcot-Marie-Tooth's atrophy has a favorable prognosis for survival.

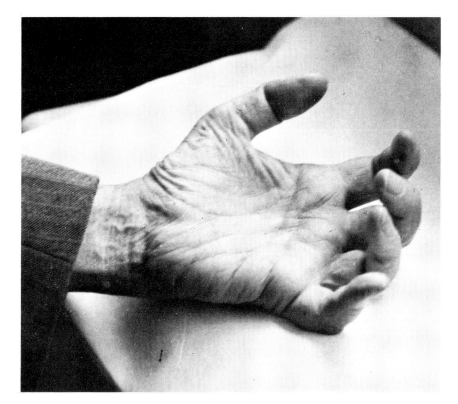

Fig. 65. Charcot-Marie-Tooth peroneal atrophy.

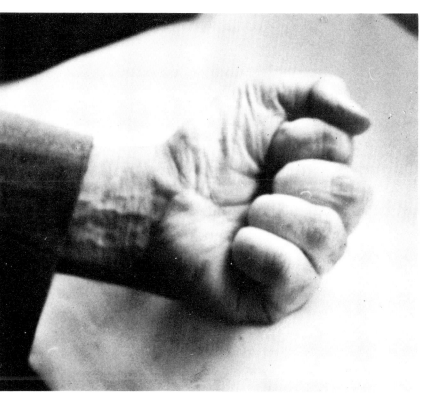

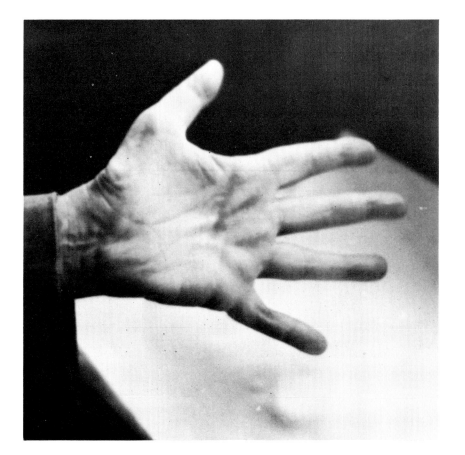

Fig. 66. Charcot-Marie-Tooth peroneal atrophy.

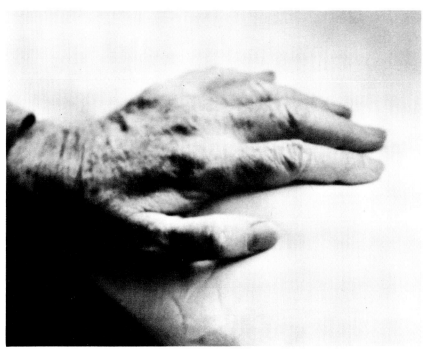

Fig. 67. Charcot-Marie-Tooth peroneal atrophy.

MONGOLISM

About 5 per cent of institutionalized mental defectives and approximately one in six or seven hundred of the general population are afflicted with mongolism. The gross morphologic appearance of the mongolian is so characteristic as to be sufficient evidence for the diagnosis. Hand formation and development in this disorder are of clinical interest and follow a readily identifiable pattern.

The hands are usually shortened, thickened and broad, with little cone-shaped fingers. The fat, flabby hand of the younger subjects has a soft and wrinkled skin on its dorsal surface, but among the older subjects the skin has become dry, rough, cold and sometimes cyanotic because of faulty local circulation. The thumb is frequently shorter than normal, and the fifth finger is curiously incurved and shortened, so that its tip may not quite reach the middle phalangeal joint of the ring finger (symptom of DuBois). Instead of the normally present two transverse palmar creases, the mongol has only one, and the curved fifth finger often presents but a single fold or crease, rather than the usual two. This anomaly follows as a consequence of the rudimentary second phalanx. Quite often other developmental defects may be found in the mongolian idiot, such as webbed fingers and toes or supernumerary digits (see *Palmar Dermatoglyphics*).

SYRINGOMYELIA

Physical findings of a characteristic type occur in the hands in syringomyelia. The essential neuropathologic features of this disease include a tubular cavitation (syrinx) of the spinal cord surrounding the central canal. Such changes are found primarily in the cervical segment of the cord, although the level of involvement is subject to wide variation. Cavity formation causes an interruption of pain and temperature fibers which decussate in the anterior commissures. As the process of destruction progresses the anterior motor horn cells of the gray cord are involved and produce the classical clinical features of syringomyelia—loss of pain and temperature sensations in the given part, and atrophy of the muscles supplied.

Fasciculations of the muscles of the hand and forearm follow anterior horn cell destruction. Bilateral, segmental loss of pain and temperature sensation occurs early, although one side is affected somewhat before the other. Touch sensation is preserved in most instances. Trophic and vasomotor disturbances are common, which account for the appearance described as "the succulent hand of

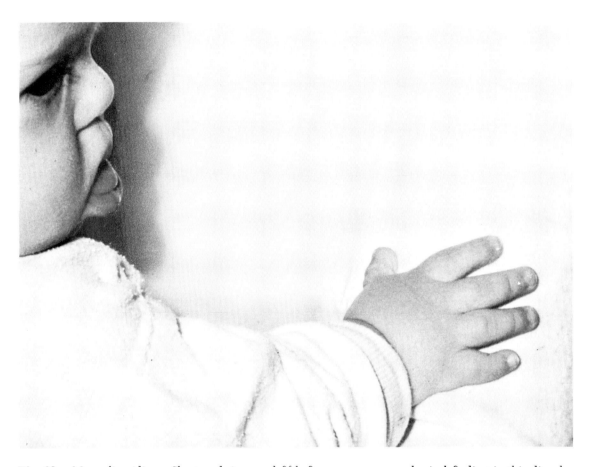

Fig. 68. Mongolian idiocy. Shortened, incurved fifth finger, a common physical finding in this disorder (symptom of DuBois).

Marinesco." The hands are livid, cold and usually wet, and the dorsum is swollen, soft and puffy ("main succulente"). Small blebs develop at the tips of the fingers. The blebs usually ulcerate and heal eventually with scar formation. Because of anesthesia in the affected areas of the hand the patient is likely to incur numerous injuries and burns, much like the traditional leper. Scars which result from bleb formation, or from frequent traumas to the hand, occasionally may hypertrophy into keloids.

Ulceration of the fingertips, whitlows and the characteristic sensory manifestations are grouped in a special form of syringomyelia known as Morvan's disease.

Severe burning pains in the hands may be a troublesome symptom ("central pains"), although pain is not a usual event in syringomyelia.

Other related phenomena may be observed in the hands of patients suffering from syringomyelia, such as thickening of the palmar aponeurosis which resembles that in Dupuytren's contracture, disturbances in the digital joints, cord arthropathies, fractures and various types of dislocations. The skin of the hand is often thin and glossy and easily injured.

In syringomyelia, as elsewhere when vasomotor and trophic disturbances are featured, hair growth in the affected parts may be arrested, or the hair may be shed. The intrinsic musculature of the hand eventually becomes severely atrophic and "claw deformity" develops gradually to maximum degree.

Weakness of the small muscles of the hand out of proportion to the degree of wasting; dissociated anesthesia (loss of heat, cold, and pain but retained sensation of light touch); the tumid, cold, wet hand; scoliosis and the shawl-distribution of neuropathologic signs should suggest the diagnosis of syringomyelia.

PINK DISEASE (Acrodynia, Swift's Disease, Erythredema)

Pink disease is of unknown cause. It affects children, usually between the ages of four months to four years. Clinical features include fever, a skin rash and polyneuritis. Among the suggested causes are viral infection, vitamin deficiency and mercury intoxication. Demyelination of peripheral nerves occurs.

About one or two weeks after onset with malaise and mild fever, a generalized erythema appears. The rash quickly fades from the rest of the body, but becomes much worse in the hands and feet, which become swollen, dusky red and itchy. The pruritus may be intolerable. Desquamation follows shortly thereafter. Photophobia, stomatitis, loss of teeth and hair, and profuse sweating are common.

Neurologic features occur at about the time that the rash is full blown. Involved muscles are weak, tender and atrophic. The tendon reflexes are lost.

Recovery usually can be expected in four to six weeks in patients with mild cases, but other subjects are less fortunate and the illness may be protracted for many months.

diseases of the CARDIOVASCULAR SYSTEM

4

The cardiologist has a readily accessible font of information in the appearance of the hand in helping him to arrive at a diagnosis of disorder in the cardiovascular system. Color and temperature are quick crude indicators of blood flow. The warm, cyanotic hand points to a systemic mechanism, while a cold cyanotic hand may suggest a local circulatory impediment. Differences in size, color, and warmth in one or more fingers or in one hand as compared with the other may indicate the presence of inequalities of blood flow at various vascular levels, such as occur in aneurysms or in abnormal arteriovenous communications.

Congenital cardiovascular anomalies, such as arteriovenous fistulas or septal defects which permit mixing of the venous and arterial streams, can cause cyanosis, clubbing of the fingers and polycythemia. Other anomalies are associated with congenital cardiac malformation in almost 20 per cent of cases. Polydactyly and syndactyly, arachnodactyly and the slender hyperextensible hand habitus are observed frequently in patients with congenitally misformed hearts. Twenty per cent of patients with pulmonic valve stenosis with reversed atrial shunts and 15 per cent of subjects of atrial septal defects demonstrate classic spider hands. Arachnodactyly, first described by Marfan in 1896, is found in the syndrome named for him, but also in sickle-cell disease, and in some instances of neurofibromatosis associated with pheochromocytosis.

Marfan's syndrome is a systemically distributed disorder but has an important cardiovascular component frequently responsible for the presence of septal defects, vascular hypoplasia, and medione-

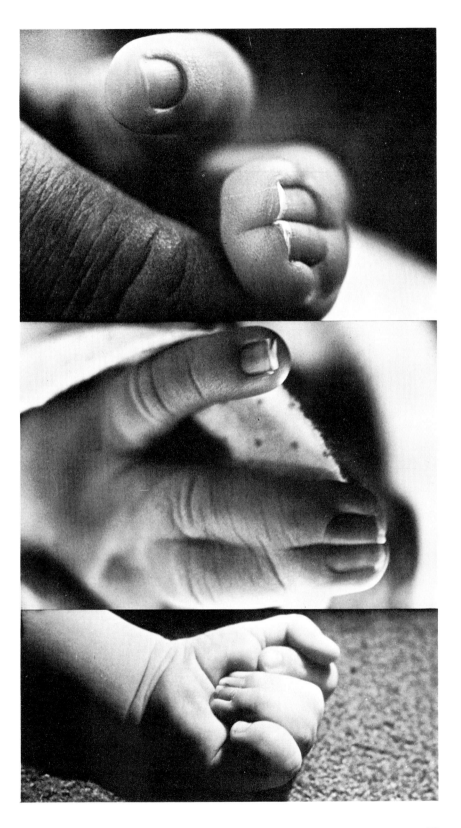

Figs. 69 & 70. Syndactyly, frequently associated with other congenital deformities, notably those which involve the cardiac structures. This child is the third generation in which syndactylism is manifest, but is otherwise normal (Courtesy of Theodore Kevin Gallagher, Los Angeles, Calif.)

Fig. 71. Syndactylism in otherwise normal infant. Father and grandparents had webbed toes. The presence of syndactylism suggests other congenital malformations, frequently involving the cardiovascular structures.

crosis of the aorta. The latter may result in aortic dissection, a not uncommon mechanism which accounts for the shortened life span expected in these subjects.

Congenital heart disease is found in about one quarter of mongolian idiots. The abnormalities include septal defects, Fallot's tetralogy and open ductus Botalli. This combination of defects produces a variety of unusual hand configurations, adding those related to the cardiac disease to the fat, soft, thin-skinned mongoloid features. Peripheral circulatory impairment is frequently present and accounts for the cold, cyanotic hand seen quite often in mongolian idiocy. Syndactyly and webbed digits are sometimes present in these patients as in many individuals with embryonic or genetic dysgerminisms.

Pocked or stippled nails have been observed in 95 per cent of subjects of acute rheumatic fever and chorea. This manifestation is probably due to a nonspecific nutritional defect. In active rheumatic fever, firm subcutaneous nodules are observed occasionally over the bony prominences of the wrist and knuckles. Hemosiderin deposits in the skin give a curious pigmented appearance to the dorsum of the hand in some children in congestive heart failure.

MYOCARDIAL INFARCTION

Several painful reflex phenomena in the upper extremity have been described as sequelae of myocardial infarction. These include the shoulder-hand syndrome, thickening of the palmar fascia, and arthralgia of the finger joints. The exact mechanisms responsible for these events are not clear, although many investigators have suggested that mediation of neurotrophic stimuli from the area of infarction to the cervical dermatomes seems most likely.

Shapiro reported an occurrence of symmetric, painless ulceration in the hands of a patient, 12 hours after the onset of acute posterior myocardial infarction. Thinly walled vesicles develop at the metacarpophalangeal joints adjacent the index fingers. The small blebs soon rupture and leave deeply punched-out ulcers which may not heal for 10 to 12 weeks. Trophic ulcerations on the hands complicating myocardial infarction are thought to be caused by impulses arising from the infarcted heart muscle and mediated through sensory nerves.

Dupuytren's contracture occurs occasionally in association with coronary artery disease, and is due to irritation of sympathetic ganglia, but, again, the mechanism is not clear. Joint swelling and pain in the fingers may be observed in patients with myocardial infarction. This may be due to a flareup of a pre-existing arthritis, or perhaps to enkindlement of a latent arthropathy of the "neurogenic" type. Postinfarctional sclerodactylia (see *Shoulder-Hand Syndrome*) is ascribed to increased vasoconstriction of peripheral arteries initiated by pain and anxiety attendant upon the cardiac disease.

Hypercholesterolemia and hyperlipemia are associated with a higher incidence of atherosclerosis and an increased tendency to coronary artery disease. When serum lipid concentrations reach a critical level, xanthomata appear on the hands, particularly in the palmar folds and in the creases of the fingers. Xanthomata have the appearance of flat, narrow tan or yellowish ribbons arranged along the creases, or as flat-topped papular lesions which represent deposits of fat in the skin.

Transverse white bands have been described in the nails of patients suffering with myocardial infarction.

SHOCK

Not only in connection with myocardial infarction, but in any clinical situation when a warm, pale hand becomes abruptly cold and cyanotic, it forebodes an extremely ominous sign. With the hippocratic facies it constitutes one of the most ancient and reliable of agonal signs. The hand of the patient in shock is cold, clammy wet and cyanotic. In congestive heart failure the veins are dark and distended, and the moons of the nails are either a reddish-purple or violet. The nail beds are a cyanotic slate-blue color.

SUBACUTE BACTERIAL ENDOCARDITIS

Careful examination of the hands of the patient with subacute bacterial endocarditis may be a rewarding diagnostic venture. Several classic physical findings, which are frequently associated with this disease, may be present. Some of the signs are considered pathognomonic. The latter statement refers to the Osler node, a disease-specific lesion which usually appears in the pads, or on the sides of the fingers, or sometimes in the thenar or hypothenar areas. Osler nodes are small, pea-sized nodules which are slightly raised and tender. Unfortunately, eponymic designations lead to confusion, particularly in the instance when Osler's nodes and Osler's disease must be differentiated. Hereditary or familial hemorrhagic telangiectasis is a much better term for the latter syndrome (see p. 135).

Neither are Osler's nodes to be confused with the Janeway lesion, another dermal phenomenon described in subacute bacterial endocarditis. The Janeway lesion is a small erythematous, reddish-purple

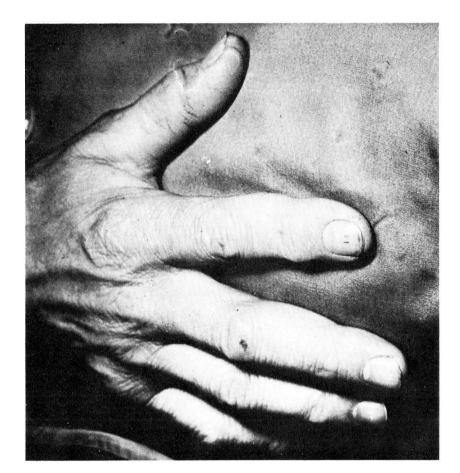

Fig. 72. Subacute bacterial endocarditis. Splinter hemorrhages under nail of index finger.

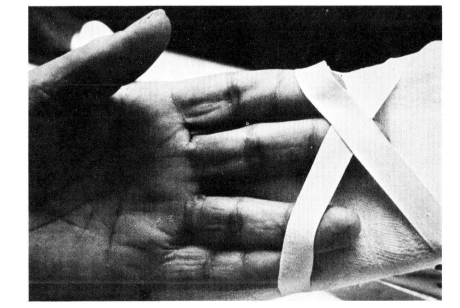

Fig. 73. Subacute bacterial endocarditis. This patient had acute bacterial endocarditis which was accompanied by generalized purpura. The major creases of the palms and fingers are a deep violet color due to purpura limited to that distribution in the hands.

or hemorrhagic patch which is somewhat nodular in form, and is found in rare instances in the palmar skin and in the sole of the foot. It is seldom tender. A few days after its onset the color of the lesion fades to a brownish hue and the irregular nodularity of the lesion gradually disappears as the skin returns to normal texture.

The Janeway lesion is more characteristic of the acute stage of bacterial endocarditis, but occasionally is present in subacute forms. However, it is another in a long list of eponymic ghosts that has been afforded extended survival by automatic inclusion in successive editions of textbooks. This phenomenon exists in the most fleeting of life spans at best, is extremely rare, and may perhaps be a vanishing entity. Dr. Bean, who has devoted a large part of his brilliant career as observer and recorder of similar cutaneous phenomena, admits having seen but one Janeway lesion in the past ten years. This exceeds by one the number most clinicians have seen.

Petechial hemorrhages in the skin and nail beds are found frequently in the hands of patients afflicted with bacterial endocarditis. Embolic effects are manifested as slightly tender, reddened or bruised spots in the fingers, nail beds or less often in the palms. Trophic disturbances such as wasting or hypoplasia may occur in the nails or in the intrinsic musculature of the hand.

Splinter hemorrhages are fine, linear, red streaks under the nail plates, usually arranged in an irregular picket near the free edge of the nail. They are specifically, but not exclusively, associated with subacute bacterial endocarditis. A large percentage of patients with trichiniasis will have splinter hemorrhages in the nail beds, as will a significant number of patients with rheumatic heart disease, even in the absence of valvular infection. Possibly a lowered vascular turgor permits development of these red fringes of hemorrhage at the distal rim of the nail bed. They are found also in hemorrhagic states and in certain deficiencies, such as scurvy. My colleagues and I have noted the presence of splinter hemorrhages in the nails of a patient with a bleeding tendency due to a blood dyscrasia.

Anemia is a common and outstanding clinical feature of bacterial endocarditis. Pallor in the skin of the palm and nail beds is noted in this disease as it is in anemias of any type. In members of the white race the creases of the palms are normally pink, but become pale or silvery white when the hemoglobin concentration falls to a level of approximately 7 grams per 100 milliliters of blood (Wintrobe).

Clubbing of the finger ends may be present in subacute bacterial endocarditis. When the patient has recovered from the bacteremia, clubbing usually recedes quite promptly.

My associates and I have observed a patient with acute bacterial endocarditis who developed a generalized purpuric rash, most prominently demonstrated in the creases of the hands. All the major palmar creases became a dark violet color simultaneously as large ecchymoses appeared in several other skin areas.

In subacute bacterial endocarditis a ball-valve thrombus may form and occlude the mitral opening. Such an obstruction can cause sudden coldness and cyanosis of the fingers with progression in some instances to produce gangrene of the digits.

AORTIC INSUFFICIENCY

Many of the characteristic physical findings to be seen in patients with aortic valve incompetence are secondary effects of disordered vascular dynamics produced by the augmented thrust of an elevated pulse pressure. One such effect of the forceful pulsation is the "Quincke pulse." This phenomenon is a visible pulsatile blushing synchronous with the heartbeat in the small vessels of the fingertip pulp and nail bed. Visualization of the throbbing color changes is facilitated by observation through a glass microscope slide which is pressed gently against the finger pad.

The same type of capillary pulsations is also found in certain other pathologic states in which a high cardiac stroke output is an associated event. A widened pulse pressure is a common denominator in patients who have high fevers, anemia, hyperthyroidism and patent ductus arteriosus. Any condition which is attended by a high pulse pressure is capable of causing capillary pulsations of the Quincke type.

Sometimes it is possible to count the pulse of a patient with an elevated pulse pressure while holding his hand during an ordinary handshake, because of the transmission of pulsations from the palms and fingers.

Another unrelated, but interesting finding in the hands of the patient with aortic insufficiency is a paradoxic palmar pallor. Even in the absence of anemia there is frequently an unexplained pallid appearance to the palm in patients with aortic valve disease. The manual laborer may exhibit yellowish or pale palms due to dense callus formations, but these hands are seldom confused with those of either the patient with anemia or one with aortic insufficiency.

SCALENUS ANTICUS AND RELATED SYNDROMES

There are several neurovascular syndromes which produce important clinical effects in the hands. The majority of these conditions derive from mechanical impediments at the root of the neck, which reduce the blood supply, or impinge on the nerves to the upper extremities. Heavy drag of the upper limb on the anatomic structures traversing the cervical triangles, amplification by pulling or stretching, and tightness of the musculature at the point of blood vessel or nerve emergence create symptomatic situations. Arterial supply to the upper extremity is channeled through a relatively crowded compartment beneath the clavicle, where the scalenus anticus muscle and the first rib provide possible restricting boundaries. The result of each of these various syndromes (scalenus anticus, thoracic outlet, costoclavicular and hyperabduction syndromes) is pain in the arm and hand, trophic changes and weakness. Paresthesias, color changes, atrophy of the intrinsic muscles of the hand, and obliteration of the radial pulse may occur in any of the above-mentioned disorders. Through sympathetic irritation a neurovascular dystrophy of the Raynaud's type may be produced.

The scalenus anticus syndrome is caused by a tightness of the scalenus anticus muscle which causes pressure on the branches of the brachial plexus as they exit beneath its edge. Painful paresthesias in the arm and hand can be reproduced by the examiner by pressing his thumb firmly against the scalene muscle group above the clavicle. Patients may volunteer the information that swinging the arms or carrying a heavy brief case or valise while walking will bring on the classic pain and paresthesias in the hand or upper extremity.

The Adson maneuver will emphasize the defect and is used to establish the role played by the scalene muscle in the symptomatology. In this test, the patient is instructed to hold his arms at the side, and extend the neck. When he takes a deep inspiration and holds it, as the chin is rotated forcibly toward the involved side, the radial pulse is shut off, and the pain and other symptoms are reproduced.

The *thoracic outlet syndrome* is due to angulation of the subclavian artery and the brachial plexus by a prominent, enlarged or abnormally situated first rib.

The *hyperabduction syndrome* is due to compression of the same neurovascular structures by hyperabduction of the upper extremity. It occurs most often during the night among people who sleep with their head resting on the hyperextended arm. Students still rather refer to this syndrome as "Saturday night palsy" or "honeymoon paralysis."

The *costoclavicular syndrome* refers to the same symptoms as those listed above, resultant from pinching of the neurovascular elements between the first rib and clavicle by any force which tends to displace the shoulder girdle downward and backward.

All of these syndromes may cause a Raynaud's phenomenon in the upper extremity. In patients with longstanding, unattended disease, thinning of the fingertip pad may occur, in addition to other physical effects of impaired arterial blood flow or nerve supply to the extremity. Such effects include coldness, loss of hair on the proximal phalanx, and color changes. Trophic ulcerations on the digits and abnormalities of the nail may be expected in advanced degrees of circulatory or nerve interference. A possible end result of these syndromes is either a spotty necrosis or a more extensive, segmental gangrene of the fingers.

Individuals who have been afflicted chronically with this type of disorder learn eventually to offset the painful pull of the arm by assuming a characteristic position in which the arms are folded across the chest at a high level and the shoulders are held hunched.

PERIPHERAL VASCULAR DISEASE

Gangrene of the fingertips may complicate numerous severe systemic infections such as meningitis, malaria, typhus fever, typhoid fever, scarlet fever, diphtheria, pneumonia and severe bacteremia. Because of their anatomic structure and organization and relatively great distance from the heart, the arteries of the hand readily reflect occlusive damage. Uncompensated block in the delivery of blood to the fingers results in color and temperature changes, slowly healing ulcerations, trophic distortions of the nails and gangrene.

Severe Raynaud's phenomenon with development of gangrenous fingertips has been reported in association with periarteritis nodosa. Digital gangrene may attend vascular interference at any level along the arterial supply line, such as occurs in some instances of aneurysm, scalenus anticus syndrome, cervical rib, or in sclerotic, spastic, embolic or thrombotic occlusive disease.

The commonest peripheral vascular diseases are arteriosclerosis and thromboangiitis obliterans, which together comprise 95 per cent of all such problems.

Arteriosclerosis is by far the most frequently encountered peripheral vascular disorder. An age-linked disease, with strong influences from nature and nurture, it is found six times more often in males than in females. Diabetics, particularly those with low insulin requirements, show an increased susceptibility, and acquire their arteriosclerotic disease at an earlier age than does the general population.

Although Buerger's disease (thromboangiitis obliterans) usually attacks vessels of the lower extremity, in about 2 per cent of the patients it may be limited to the upper extremity alone, and in another 25 per cent, both hands and feet are involved. Migratory,

Fig. 74. Gangrene of the hand in arteriosclerotic obliterative vascular disease.

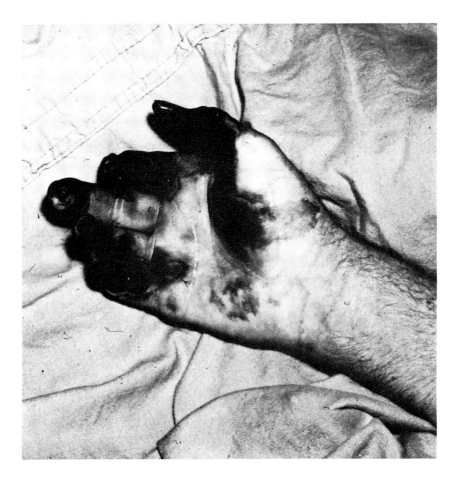

superficial thrombophlebitis is a sentinel finding in about 70 per cent of individuals with Buerger's disease. Jewish males in their middle years of life are particularly susceptible, and cold weather and tobacco are prominent trigger factors.

Arteriovenous aneurysms or fistulas in the upper extremity are either congenital or acquired. Congenital fistulas are the result of defective evolution during the transition between primitive and adult vascular patterns. Their presence may be suspected when there is an increased limb length on one side, or a unilateral enlargement of the hand, or perhaps a part of the hand. Color changes are often present, and the degree of duskiness or plethora depends upon the grade of abnormalcy in vascular communications. An increase in skin temperature in the hand is readily detectable, and a continuous murmur is audible over varicose vessels which may be present.

It is suggested that the hands of the patient offer to the examiner a readily accessible source of clinical information in many different bodily systems. By virtue of their usual state of nakedness and the anatomically peninsular situation, the hands have an important heat-regulatory function. Heat loss through the rich vascular networks of the hand has been a recent target of interest and investigation by physiologists concerned with human thermodynamics. A crude index of changes in the arterial wall throughout the general circulation can be estimated by observation of vascular integrity and behavior of digital vessels. From a practical standpoint, this estimation is possible by a bedside or office examination, largely by inspection of skin and nail color, and by the temperature of the hand. Mottled, blotchy, pale or dusky hands indicate neurovascular instability, or can denote more serious vascular inadequacy when trophic disturbances are also present.

Atrophy or dystrophy are most likely to show in the nails first by the presence of irregularities of configuration and growth. Nails become split at the ends, or laminated (onychoschizia) and lose the normal contour of their surfaces and develop crinkled, shingled edges. Growth of nails and hair on the dorsum of the hands and the proximal phalanges is retarded. As arterial flow is compromised further, the fleshy pads at the ends of the fingers become thinned, cold and pale, and eventually painful blisters form. Ulcerations and dark, ominous spots appear as gangrene begins.

One of the many uses of the opening handshake with the patient is in the appreciation of the "feel" of the hand—the texture and temperature of the skin. It is impossible to come away from the ancient custom of shaking hands with a person without acquiring some information of clinical value.

Use of other diagnostic implements for closer identification of subtle or obscure vascular diseases may be required, to be sure. An oscillometer and thermocouple permits quantitative confirmation of what most clinicians had already ascertained. But the first clues in generalized peripheral vascular disease are present in the hands in many instances, and perception of these indicators (temperature and color) does not ordinarily require the use of special diagnostic instruments.

RAYNAUD'S DISEASE

Raynaud's disease is a vasospastic disorder which occurs most often in young, hypometabolic women during the child-bearing years. It is idiopathic, bilateral, symmetric and paroxysmal, and characteristically is produced by arteriolar and arterial contraction of digital vessels, triggered by exposure of the parts to cold. Fatigue, imbibing hot or cold liquids and emotional stresses are secondary factors which augment the local vascular sensitivity and induce paroxysms.

During an attack the tips of the fingers or the entire digit become suddenly pale to dead white and cool. Subjectively the patient experiences pain and tingling in the affected parts of the fingers, and diminished capacity for fine movements. Paresthesias alter perceptive acuity sufficiently to cause the individual to experience transient difficulty in picking up small objects. Subsequent vasodilatation follows, sensation and warmth returns and the fingers become dusky or cyanotic and sweaty. Finally a hyperemic phase develops, with redness and a sensation of burning and tightness in the fingers. Occasionally only two of these stages are present, with cyanosis or pallor progressing directly to rubor. The duration of the paroxysm is variable, from minutes to hours.

Raynaud's phenomenon is the term applied to these same paroxysmal vasospasms in the hands, when they occur secondarily to certain systemic diseases. Some of the possible "primary" conditions are scleroderma, systemic lupus erythematosus, dermatomyositis and peripheral vascular disease. This phenomenon has been found in association with cervical rib, or tumors which caused pressure on the brachial plexus, and in instances of encroachment by aneurysm within the thorax. Periarteritis nodosa, Buerger's disease and post-traumatic states have been responsible etiologically in the production of Raynaud's phenomenon.

More than half of a large series of patients with Raynaud's phenomenon reported by de Takats had a collagen disorder of one kind or another. Most often the associated dyscollagenosis was scleroderma. By the time it is fully developed, scleroderma does not con-

Fig. 75. Raynaud's phenomenon. Vasospastic, trophic changes of the hands manifest by dryness, cracking, fissures and early ulceration of fingertips.

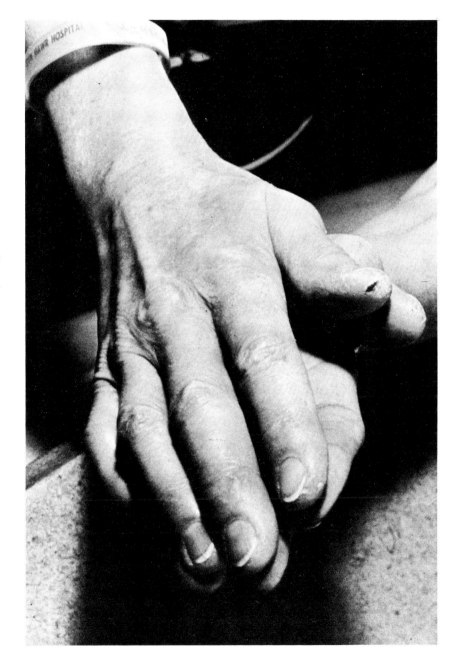

tinue to manifest the color changes characteristic of Raynaud's phenomenon. That is to say that advanced scleroderma has gotten beyond the point of going through the usual color sequence. Even excluding the late cases of scleroderma from the statistics, half of the remainder were incipient or latent stages which showed typic Raynaud's vasospasm. Of special interest is the interval between the development of Raynaud's phenomenon and the diagnosis of scleroderma, which ranged from three to 16 years. Only half of the cases were diagnosed within two years of the onset of Raynaud's phenomenon. This information makes one question the accuracy of a diagnosis of *primary* Raynaud's disease. Formerly the criteria for labeling the condition as primary, rather than secondary, was the failure to demonstrate a causative underlying disorder within a two-year period. Perhaps we have been caught up in a snarl of semantics, and the need for redundant and overlapping terminology has disappeared in the light of newer knowledge and longer follow-up.

Scleroderma is by far the most frequently occurring collagen disease related to the presence of Raynaud's phenomenon, but systemic lupus erythematosus and dermatomyositis are also causally associated.

A third of de Takats' patients had peripheral vascular disease as an underlying mechanism. These individuals suffered from vascular disorders related to frostbite, embolus, thromboangiitis, rheumatic arteritis and atherosclerosis. Other less common primary factors are autonomic hyperactivity, polycythemia vera, and pulmonary hypertension. In a small percentage of patients, cold agglutinins or cryoglobulins are demonstrable.

In patients with chronic cases, thinning and tapering of the pulp of the fingertips occur. Nails tend to grow more slowly than normally because of the localized nutritional deficit. The fingernails are frequently curved longitudinally. Also related to circulatory impairment, ulcerated blebs may develop on the digits, which heal subsequently with the formation of silvery, stellate scars. Between attacks the fingers are usually redder than normal.

In Raynaud's phenomenon and several other vasospastic conditions such as scleroderma, an extensive pterygium may develop. This is a thin, arciform shelf or fold of pale tissue which obliterates the normally distinct boundaries between the nail fold and cuticle, and between the cuticle and nail plate. Retarded growth of nails, thickening and claw-nail deformity may be anticipated in digits in which arterial insufficiency exists. Hair growth, normally present on the dorsum of the proximal phalanges, will be sparse or absent in the fingers whenever local arterial inadequacy occurs from any mechanism. If circulatory interference is severe enough, gangrene of the fingers can occur, beginning as usual at the tips.

In spite of the difficulty in separating primary Raynaud's disease from secondary Raynaud's phenomenon in some instances, there are certain clinical differences that may aid in arriving at a correct diagnosis. Raynaud's disease is usually symmetric. There is frequently an hereditary factor and the disease is progressive, up to the point of gangrene and severe atrophic changes. Raynaud's phenomenon, however, is not often symmetric and it is nonprogressive. Hereditary influences are not apparent in Raynaud's phenomenon.

ERYTHROMELALGIA

Erythromelalgia, described by Weir Mitchell, is a vasomotor disturbance that has many clinical features which places it in a diametrically opposite position from that of Raynaud's disease. In its idiopathic form there are paroxysms of bilateral vasodilatation. It occurs also as a secondary effect in several systemic diseases.

It is characterized by an increased skin temperature and redness of the hands (or feet) which are accompanied by severe painful burning or tingling sensations in the hyperemic areas. Attacks are precipitated by excitement or by subjecting the sensitive extremities to environmental temperatures in excess of their individual critical level. Sometimes this temperature may be no higher than that produced by wearing heavy socks or gloves, or by covering with ordinary bedclothing. Warm summer weather may be sufficient to induce a paroxysm. Arterial pulsations are bounding in character, and the hands appear constantly intensely reddened or purplish. The veins on the dorsum of the hand appear fully distended. Holding the hands in a dependent position may sometimes precipitate an episode or intensify the burning paresthesias. Cooling the affected parts, or elevating them, eases the discomfort, and patients quickly learn that the symptoms can be relieved by immersing their hands in ice water.

Occasionally, erythromelalgia is found in association with hypertensive cardiovascular disease, gout, diabetes mellitus, rheumatoid arthritis, arteriosclerosis obliterans and thromboangiitis obliterans. It is frequently encountered in polycythemia, both primary and secondary. The latter etiologic relationship is particularly prominent in hypoxic (chronic pulmonary disease) polycythemia.

ACROCYANOSIS

Differentiation of erythromelalgia and acroparesthesia from acrocyanosis should not be difficult. Acrocyanosis resembles Raynaud's disease somewhat, in that there appears to be an increased arteriolar tonus in the vessels of the skin, especially those in the hands, and to a lesser degree in the feet.

The hands in acrocyanosis are constantly cold, cyanotic and sweaty. When the parts are exposed to cold the symptoms are accentuated, with intensification of the blueness beginning at the wrist and progressing toward the fingertips. Involved fingers appear swollen but pain is not a prominent feature, and trophic changes or gangrene do not occur.

CLUBBING OF THE FINGERS

From the earliest days of medical record it has been known that in certain disease states the fingertips become thickened in all diameters, and the nails exhibit an exaggerated curving in both directions, axially and from side to side. Bulbous expansion of the terminal phalanx is observed in several clinical situations, to the delight of every instructor in physical diagnosis and his pupils. It is a dramatic physical sign with a nicely correlated physiologic mechanism.

Clubbing of the fingers is always accompanied by an increase in blood flow through the enlarged phalanx. In the normal digit the gradient of blood pressure diminishes progressively toward the distal end, but in the presence of clubbing this does not occur.

From an etiologic standpoint, there are two general types of clubbing, which differ significantly from each other in their appearance. A dusky, richly vascular variety, frequently accompanied by a reddish-brown pigmentation of the skin proximal to the lunule, is more likely to be found in association with congenital, cyanotic cardiac disease. Histologically this type of clubbing is secondary to increased vascularity, vasodilatation, and augmented delivery of blood to the fingertips.

Another major type of clubbing has a drier, more pallid, less engorged appearance because the enlargement of the distal phalanx is composed mainly of connective tissue overgrowth between the nail plate and the bone. Chronic pulmonary disease is more often the underlying defect responsible for the formation of this type of clubbing.

Clubbing may be present in a single digit or in several fingers. Sometimes it affects one limb, but more frequently is a bilateral finding. Unilateral clubbing may occur when the appropriate error in circulatory dynamics is limited to the vasculature supplying one extremity. Clubbing in only one limb has been demonstrated in an arteriovenous communication, with increased venous pressure, such

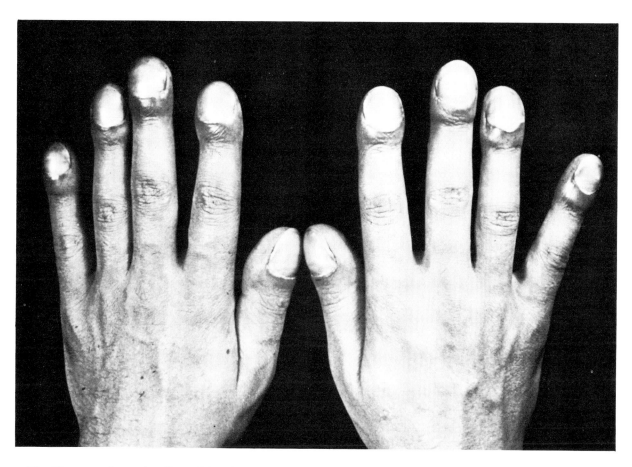

Fig. 76. Tetralogy of Fallot. Clubbed fingers in cyanotic, congenital heart disease. Note pigmentation of the tissues proximal to the nail fold. This type of pigmentation is not usually seen in clubbing due to chronic pulmonary disease.

Fig. 77. Pulmonary fibrosis. In chronic lung disease, "beaking" of the nail may occur. This appears as an exaggerated convexity of the nail surface, and represents a lesser magnitude of change than that seen in the fully developed clubbing deformity.

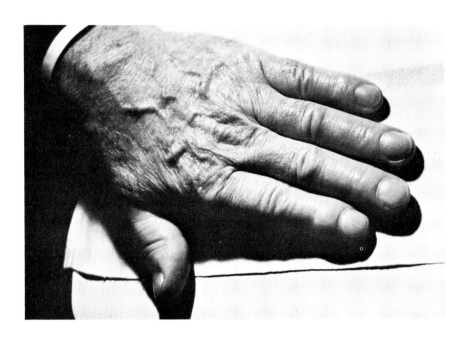

Fig. 78. "Murderer's thumbs." Wide, short thumb nail and blunted tip, seen in certain endocrinopathies such as acromegaly and cretinism, but often in normal people as an heritable trait.

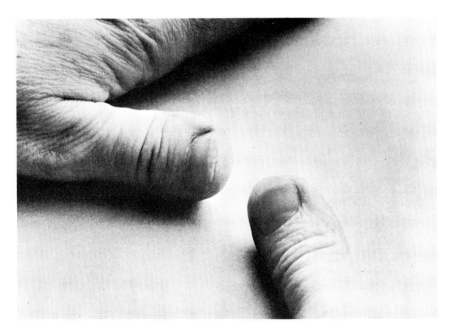

as occurs in thrombosis of the axillary vein, or with aneurysmal dilatation of the aortic arch. Aneurysm of the subclavian artery on the same side can cause unilateral clubbing of the fingers.

Arteriovenous mixing in congenital heart disease causes cyanosis in the skin and mucous membranes, especially prominent in the fingertips and nail beds. The cyanosis thus produced occurs first and subsequently is followed by the clubbing phenomenon. Neither cyanosis nor clubbing, however, develops usually before the subject reaches the age of two years. Clubbing of fingers in congenital cardiac defects occurs initially in the index finger and thumb and later advances to involve all of the fingers. It disappears promptly after surgical correction of the abnormal course of blood circulation.

In the child with clubbed fingers who does not have cyanosis, a congenital cardiac malformation is extremely unlikely, and an extracardiac cause must be sought. There is a direct relationship between the degree of polycythemia and the severity of the clubbing deformity.

Whenever one congenital developmental error is encountered it is well to look for others, since multiple embryologic defects are the rule. Accessory nipple, polydactyly and syndactyly are found frequently in association with congenital heart disease (see *Palmar Dermatoglyphics*).

Care must be exercised in the interpretation of clubbing of the fingers in the occasional healthy teen-aged male who may show this phenomenon as a normal, transient, familial variant.

In sarcoidosis a single digital tip may be enlarged and flattened front to back.

In other cardiocirculatory diseases in which anoxia is a feature, clubbing of the digits is a possible associated finding. Within this category are those congenital cardiac defects which cause cyanosis and polycythemia, such as in right-to-left, or venous-to-arterial, intracardiac or extracardiac shunt (e.g., tetralogy of Fallot).

Rouleaux formation of erythrocytes reduces the area of diffusion surfaces in the blood cell and thereby causes a relative tissue anoxia. Therefore, in diseases in which there is an increase in serum globulin concentrations, and consequent exaggerated rouleaux formation, the digits may exhibit clubbing. Clubbing occurs sometimes in anoxic states produced by hemoglobinemia.

Apart from the more common cardiopulmonary causes, the hand of certain individuals with sprue, parasitic infestation, cirrhosis (particularly of the biliary type), amebic and bacillary dysentery, chronic nephritis, myxedema, Raynaud's phenomenon, ulcerative colitis and subacute bacterial endocarditis may demonstrate clubbed fingers.

A bulbous type of clubbing occurs in hypoparathyroidism, due to resorption of the distal phalanges (vide supra).

Minor changes in the contour of the distal phalanx (such as slight downward cowling or "beaking" of the nail) may be representative of an early stage of clubbing. This may progress eventually to the full-blown clubbed-finger deformity, but more often represents an end-stage effect. Increased convexity of the entire nail surface, sometimes referred to as a "watch-crystal deformity," is seen in some instances of Laennec's cirrhosis.

Hippocratic fingers have an ancient heritage in physical diagnosis, and refer to the bulb-like enlargement of the distal phalanges seen in some cases of chronic pulmonary tuberculosis. The nails are bowed boldly over the ends of the fingers, covering at least half of the tips. The nail beds are full and usually pale, and there is no noticeable pigmentation in the adjacent cuticle.

In instances when the underlying causative process is interrupted, and normal physiologic relationships have been restored by appropriate therapy, the clubbing phenomenon can be seen to stop. As nail growth thereafter proceeds in a normal way a distinct line of transition can be seen in the nail plate. This has the appearance of a definite groove which marks the point at which the disease process had ended. The new nail eventually grows out and effaces the transverse groove of demarcation.

PULMONARY HYPERTROPHIC OSTEOARTHROPATHY
(Marie-Bamberger Syndrome)

Enlargement of the distal ends of the extremities occurs as part of the Marie-Bamberger syndrome, as an effect of a curious neural reflex related to intrathoracic disease. It has been shown that the afferent impulses may originate in the pleural surfaces, and travel along the vagus nerve. Clubbing of the digits may or may not be a part of the physical changes in the distal third of the extremity. The swelling involves the lower ends of the bones of the forearm and wrist. The enlargement is usually warm and painful, and is made up of connective tissue overgrowth which takes place above the periosteum, and new bone formation beneath it. Joint spaces are not affected but a periarthritis is identifiable on biopsy study.

Included among the causes of this type of change in the extremities are such pulmonary disorders as bronchiectasis, tuberculosis, abscess of the lung and pulmonic hemangiomata.

This phenomenon constitutes an interesting and valuable sign in neoplastic disease, either primary or metastatic. It may be one of

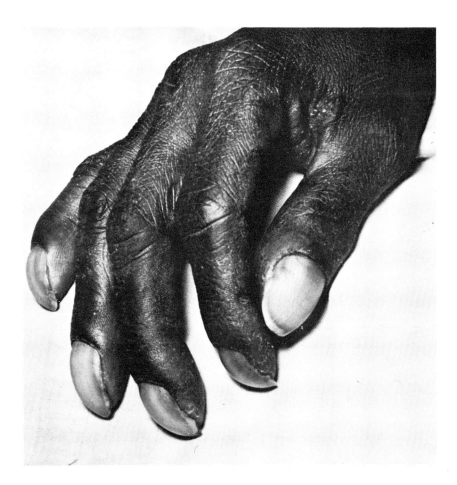

Fig. 79. Cystic disease of the lungs—clubbed fingers.

the earliest physical clues to appear. Pain in the distal joints and swelling of soft tissues are relieved dramatically and suddenly by section of the vagus nerve as it enters the hilum of the lung. Remission of symptoms is possible even if the tumor is allowed to remain in place. Similarly, relief of symptoms is achieved by surgical removal of the primary or secondary tumor of the lung, or when the vagus nerve is severed during surgery.

5 *disorders of* METABOLISM

GOUT

Although gout characteristically affects the metatarsophalangeal joints, especially of the great toe (podagra) in about 50 per cent of the cases, the hand may be the site of tophaceous deposits and arthritic manifestations due to this disease. Urate crystals may collect in nodular enlargements of the metacarpophalangeal joints or at the interphalangeal joints, producing deformity, stiffness, and interference with flexion. Unless an acute gouty arthritis is accompanied by classic signs of local heat and redness, the tophaceous nodules are not usually tender. As the tophus becomes larger the overlying skin is thin and stretched by the enlarging masses and spontaneous rupture of the nodule may occur. An ulcerated area develops and eventually a sinus tract forms from the tophus to the skin surface and exudes a white chalky crystalline material made up of urate. This is pathognomonic of gout.

Extremes of distortion result from the grotesque knobby masses that develop in the periarticular tissues. Crippling disfigurement of the hand may occur, even to the point of complete incapacitation. Crowding of the hand by large gnarled, misshaped fingers, studded with tophi and multiple discharging sinuses offers a grave threat to circulatory integrity. To relieve the circulatory or mechanical effects of disease it may be necessary ultimately to accede to the therapy of defeat—amputation of one or more digits.

Frequently, gout may be present as an additional metabolic error in persons who suffer from other forms of chemical or collagenous tissue disorders.

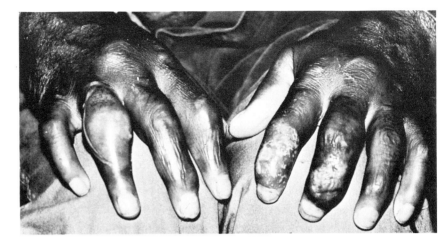

Fig. 80. Gout.

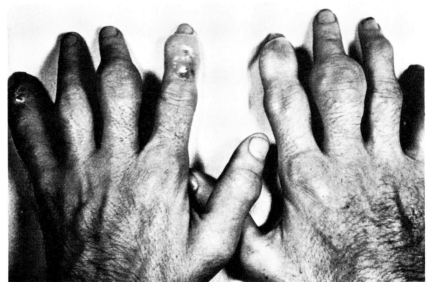

Fig. 81. Gout. Arthritic deformity and tophaceous deposits in digits. Ulceration and sinus formation has occurred with the discharge of urate-containing material.

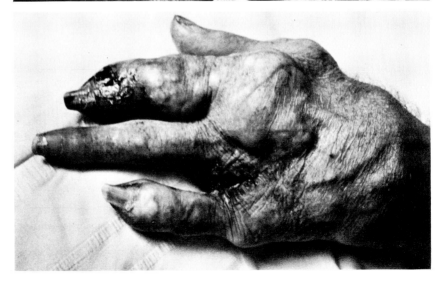

Fig. 82. Gout. Tophaceous nodules, ulcerations, and severe gouty arthritic deformity. Ring finger has been amputated because of extensive destructive effects of advanced disease.

DIABETES MELLITUS

The patient with diabetes mellitus demonstrates several physical effects of metabolic derangement in his hand. One of these signs is the occurrence of xanthomas on the palmar surfaces, generally distributed along the creases of the fingers and palms and in the webbing of the digits.

Xanthomas are small, superficial yellow or tan papules, strips or nodules which represent fatty deposition in the skin. They may be accompanied by intense itching, secondary excoriation, and infection. Or they may present as inflammatory processes affecting the subcutaneous tissues. The tendency to the formation of xanthomas in the diabetic is a reflection of disturbance of lipid metabolism which is characteristic in this disease. By projection of this relationship we may anticipate the formation of xanthomatosis in many other systemic metabolic diseases in which high concentrations of fat occur in the serum. Such is, in fact, the case in obstructive jaundice, biliary cirrhosis, and in certain hormonal imbalances of pancreatic, thyroid, and gonadal function in which lipid levels are increased to a threshold concentration. A high level of serum lipids, approximately 1800 milligrams per 100 milliliters, is required to reach that which is likely to be threshold for the formation of fatty tumors in the skin. It is interesting to note that xanthomas will disappear if hyperlipemia is reduced to a critical level at about 1800 milligrams per 100 milliliters or less.

Xanthoma diabeticorum is a somewhat rare cutaneous complication of diabetes. It features the development of small, discrete nodules, ranging in size from 1 to 3 millimeters in diameter, which stud the skin overlying the knees, elbows, forearms, buttocks, and the back of the hand. These lesions are hard, raised and non-tender. The summit of the nodule is usually yellow or light tan in color, darkening to a reddish-brown at the base. The presence of xanthoma diabeticorum in the diabetic is suggestive of hypercholesterolemia and poor metabolic control of the disease. Disappearance of the xanthomas may be expected upon correction of these conditions.

Occasionally a pellagroid pigmentation of the skin of the diabetic's hand may occur, with atrophy of the skin and a predilection to the development of senile purpura.

The well-known predisposition to infection among diabetics may be responsible for the increased tendency to the formation of paronychia and other evidences of cutaneous and subcutaneous infection, including the dreaded carbuncle on the dorsum of the hand. Moreover, these infections tend to heal more slowly than in the non-diabetic individual.

Fig. 83. Flat xanthomata in diabetes mellitus—thin, yellowish-tan ribbons of xanthomata distributed in the creases of fingers and palm.

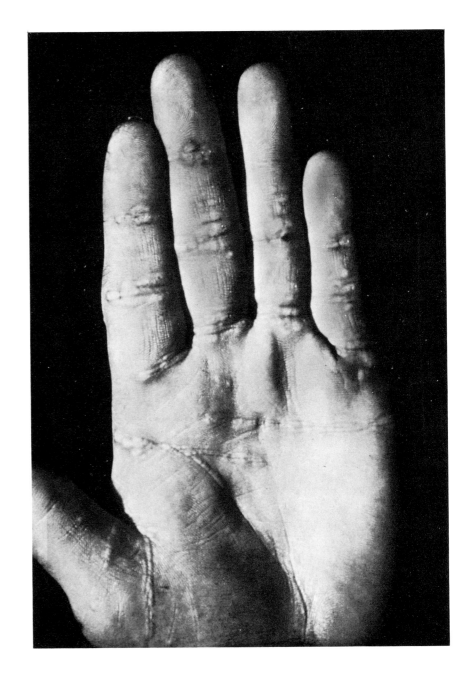

Dupuytren's contracture is somewhat more prevalent among diabetic individuals than in the general population.

The same formation of fatty tumors occurs in the skin as in the classic lipodystrophies such as in Hand-Schüller-Christian disease, Gaucher's disease, and Niemann-Pick's disease. For the most part the latter disorders show a variety in the distribution of xanthomas in the skin, especially prominent along the extensor surfaces of the body.

PORPHYRIA

There are two major clinical forms of porphyria, the erythropoietic or congenital and the hepatic or delayed. Photosensitivity, a prominent feature of porphyria, accounts for the appearance of characteristic dermal signs in the hands.

The rarer, erythropoietic type, is a metabolic defect traceable to the erythrocytic formative elements in the marrow, where faulty heme synthesis results in an overproduction of porphyrins. Massive porphyrinuria ensues and the first sign evident is the passage of red urine. Photosensitivity and its cutaneous effects may be minimal in the neonatal period and may only become symptomatic as exposure to sunlight occurs. In this disorder, as in many others dependent upon exposure of skin surfaces to sunlight or other climatic factors, the hand is the major target for dermatologic manifestations. In congenital porphyria, vesicular or bullous eruptions appear on the face, dorsum of the hand, and other exposed parts. The vesicles contain a serous fluid which usually demonstrates a red fluorescence. After rupture they heal slowly and leave depressed pigmented scars. Occasionally they become infected secondarily and angry ulcerations develop which ultimately produce severe scarring deformities, especially on the tips of the fingers. Because of the chronicity of this disorder, repeated attacks are to be expected, so that mutilation may occur. Scarring contractures of the face occur and parts of digits are often lost over the years as attack follows attack. With so dramatic an array of physical findings in the completely developed clinical picture—red urine, red or brown teeth (erythrodontia), splenomegaly, hemolytic anemia and ulcerations of the hand and face which fluoresce—diagnosis is seldom difficult.

Hepatic forms are more frequently encountered. In contrast to the congenital type, there is no hematologic disorder. Hepatic function, however, is frequently impaired and the liver constantly exhibits high concentrations of porphyrins and porphyrin precursors.

Varieties of pure and mixed forms of porphyria exist so that termi-

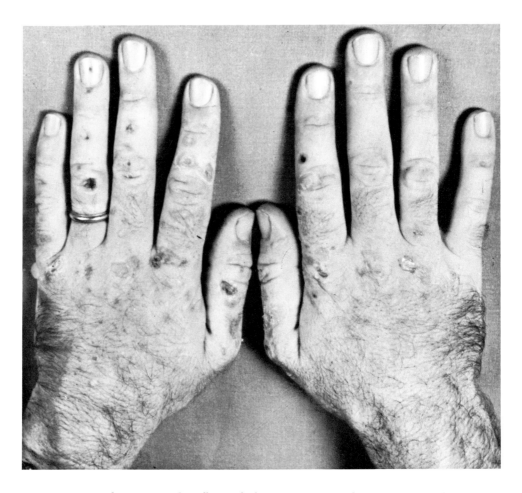

Fig. 84. Porphyria. Note the effects of photosensitivity as demonstrated in the hand of the patient with porphyria. Blisters which rupture and form shallow crusted ulcerations are common in the exposed portion of the skin, especially on dorsum of the hand. (Courtesy of J. Haserick, M.D., Cleveland Clinic, Cleveland, Ohio.)

nology becomes somewhat confused. Latent types may be triggered into acute activity by the administration of pharmaceutical agents such as barbiturates, sulfonamides and certain anesthetics.

Mild effects may be noted in certain people who show only hypersensitivity to exposure of the skin to sun from which they tend to develop small ulcerations of the skin on the dorsum of the hand and small, dense, white circular scars from previous ulcerative experiences.

WILSON'S DISEASE (Hepatolenticular Degeneration)

Symmetric basal ganglia degeneration, hepatic cirrhosis, and a greenish-brown pigmented ring on the edge of the cornea (Kayser-Fleischer) are the characteristic features of hepatolenticular degeneration or Wilson's disease. The clinical effects of this disorder proceed from an inherited abnormality in the transport of serum copper. Deposits of copper occur in the brain, kidney, and cornea, and the excretion of copper in the urine is excessive.

A most interesting observation was made by Bearn and McKusick who added another physical finding resultant from abnormal deposition of copper in the fingernail. Copper collects in the germinal end of the fingernail and imparts an "azure blue" tint to the lunula.

Phenolphthalein, a drug used frequently in proprietary laxative preparations, is also capable of producing a dark-blue discoloration of the lunula. (See also discussion of Wilson's disease on page 69 and Fig. 55.)

DEFICIENCY STATES

RICKETS

Rickets is a deficiency disease which features disturbances in calcium and phosphorus relationships. It is due to an insufficient supply of vitamin D or to inadequate sunshine.

Earliest effects of rickets are noted in the wrist owing to bilateral symmetric involvement of the epiphyseal plates which become thickened and flare out, producing a characteristic enlargement. In the acute phase of rickets the fingers participate in the generalized constitutional disturbance and are distorted by swelling which does not include the joints. This produces a sausage-shaped swelling of the shafts of the proximal and middle phalanges with a narrow-waisted configuration at the joints, the so-called "beading" of the fingers.

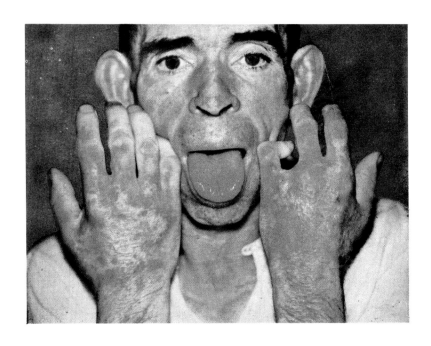

Fig. 85. Pellagra. Glossitis and pellagrous skin changes in the hands, face and exposed parts of the neck. (Courtesy of Ormsby and Montgomery: Diseases of the Skin, 7th ed. Lea & Febiger.)

PELLAGRA

Several systemic disorders have cutaneous manifestations which not infrequently involve the exposed parts of the skin surface. For that matter, a large percentage of the dermatologists' diagnoses can be made by an inspection of the patients' hands alone. Pellagra is one of these diseases.

Owing to a deficiency of niacin, one of the B-complex vitamins, pellagra affects several bodily systems and causes the characteristic "sun-burned" inflammatory lesions of the exposed skin. At first a brilliant-red macular eruption develops which most often affects the dorsum of the hands bilaterally and symmetrically, and which later worsens to appear as a shaggy inflamed scaling dermatitis. The affected portions of the skin are usually clearly demarcated from the normal skin. Vesiculation, bullae formation, ecchymoses, and dark pigmentary changes ensue in sequence. The skin rash is complicated quite often by secondary infection. After treatment with the lacking vitamin, the lesions heal ultimately with the formation of parched cicatrices.

The gauntlet distribution of the eruption, combined with glossitis and gastrointestinal symptoms, occurring usually in the warm months of the year in a nutritionally deficient population, makes diagnosis fairly easy. Chronic pellagrous changes include thickening and scaling of the skin, hyperkeratinization, and a dirty-brownish pigmentation.

Whenever symmetric cutaneous disorders are observed, a systemic etiologic mechanism, rather than a purely local one, is suggested.

XANTHOMATOSIS

Xanthomas, which appear throughout the skin in the body, are made up of lipid deposits, a scattering of giant cells, and the characteristic "xanthoma cells." They may appear in several different forms, either as flat plates or plaques or as nodular or papular lesions. They are usually non-tender and vary in size from a millimeter in diameter up to several centimeters. They are commonly yellow or orange, but may be pink or some shade of red and, in some rare instances, may be brown or tan.

The flat variety, also called xanthelasma, is frequently seen in the skin around the eyes or eyelids, but may also appear in the creases of the palm. It is seldom, if ever, seen elsewhere. The flat xanthoma is the most common of all the varieties of xanthomas and in about one quarter of the individuals with this type of lesion the serum cholesterol, esters and phospholipids are elevated. In younger

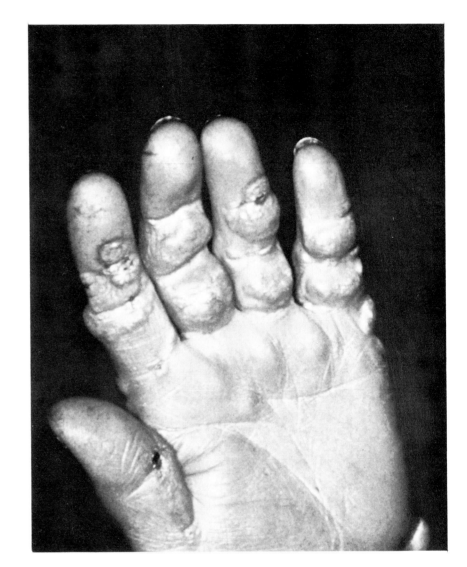

Fig. 86. Xanthomata in biliary cirrhosis. Large tuberous xanthomata in the creases of the fingers in a patient with biliary cirrhosis and extremely high level of serum cholesterol.

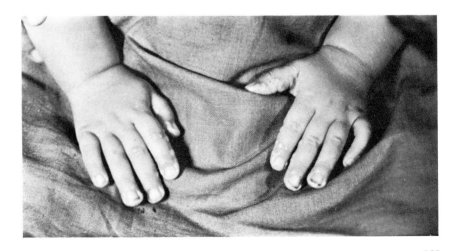

Fig. 87. Choledochal cyst. Xanthomatous infiltrations in the fingers of a child with high serum lipid concentration and choledochal cyst. (Couresy of Sidney Q. Cohlan and Herbert J. Rayden: Amer. J. Med. Vol. 32, June 1962.)

individuals its appearance may be an indication of familial hyper-cholesterolemia.

Xanthoma tuberosum is a more nodular or knobby type of xanthoma and is usually found over various areas in the body subject to pressures such as the knuckles, elbows, knees, and similar locations. The tuberous type of xanthoma is usually associated with some form of systemic dyslipidosis. The color is usually a pinkish- or yellowish-orange and varies according to the age of the lesion and its fat content. Sometimes these fatty tumors on the hands may be disfiguring and disabling.

Occasionally, xanthomas may occur as a widely disseminated papular lesion, the so-called eruptive form, and are generally extremely itchy. This type is also associated with systemic lipodystrophic conditions. Eruptive xanthomas are found in myxedema and in association with moderately elevated cholesterol levels (300 to 500 milligrams per 100 milliliters of blood serum).

Small deposits resembling xanthomas may appear in scars in certain tumors, and in areas of trauma. Fatty deposits of this sort are seen in necrobiosis lipoidica diabeticorum.

A generalized xanthomatosis is seen in many patients with biliary cirrhosis. This is usually associated with a progressively deepening jaundice and astronomic levels of serum cholesterol and phospholipids. In some instances the serum cholesterol may rise to 1000 milligrams per 100 milliliters or more. There is a marked tendency among patients with biliary cirrhosis to form plaques of xanthomatous material in the palms and around the eyelids. Papular xanthomas may be scattered widely over the remainder of the body in these patients.

Xanthochromia or xanthosis occurs when carotene or other lipochromes accumulate in the skin. This condition is quite prevalent in the diabetic individual, as has been discussed under *Diabetes Mellitus*, and appears as a peachy yellow discoloration of the palms of the hands, the soles of the feet, and on the face where the skin is thinnest. Xanthosis is sometimes confused with jaundice but is easily separable from that condition. The sclerae are not discolored in xanthosis and the serum bilirubin concentration is not elevated.

In the nephrotic syndrome, renal damage allows for a loss of serum protein which causes a mobilization of the fat stores of the body. As serum lipids increase, xanthomas may occur, but usually tend to be small and few in number.

Secondary hyperlipemia occurs sometimes in patients having chronic pancreatitis. This may produce eruptive xanthomas in the hands and elsewhere in the skin surface. Eruptive xanthomas may also be seen in von Gierke's disease. The administration of cobaltous

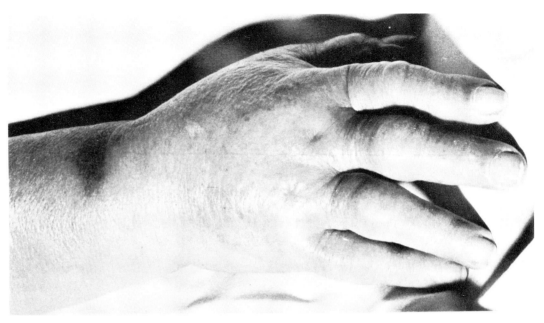

Fig. 88. Hepatic cirrhosis. Edema of the hand and ecchymosis in a patient who has severe hepatic cirrhosis, hypoproteinemia, and generalized anasarca.

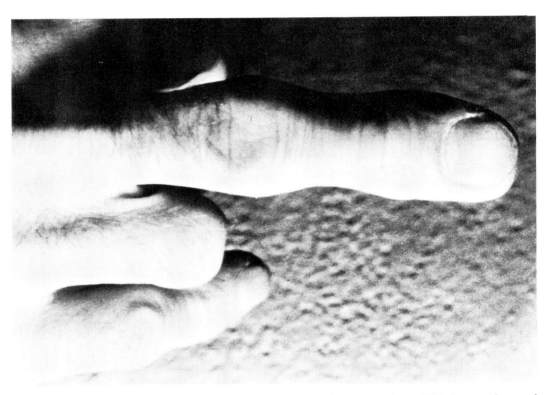

Fig. 89. Hepatic cirrhosis. Flattened nails may occur in hepatic cirrhosis. This is one of several effects, such as white nails, convex nails and beaking or clubbing that occur in patients with cirrhosis. This patient also demonstrates a thickened middle phalangeal joint due to hypertrophic arthritis.

chloride has been found to increase the level of serum lipids. This is due to a decrease in metabolism by a cobalt-induced goiter. Xanthomas have been associated with the increase in lipid levels under these circumstances.

HEPATIC CIRRHOSIS

Hormonal imbalance and nutritional deficits are responsible for many of the physical signs encountered in the patient with hepatic cirrhosis. Other visible effects are related to disturbances of pigment metabolism and to vascular abnormalities.

Certain noteworthy effects of the various metabolic disorders are present quite often in the hands of cirrhotic patients. The structure and appearance of the fingernails, in particular, undergo changes which are not altogether specific nor necessarily diagnostic of cirrhosis, but represent rather interesting characteristics of secondary importance in the clinical picture. In some individuals the fingernails may be exceptionally flat while in others they may be inordinately convex. Occasionally, the surface of the nail is convex and the distal edge of the nail is cowled over the ends of the fingertips, the so-called "watch crystal" nail, a configuration which resembles an inverted shallow bowl.

Palmar erythema is a classic physical feature in hepatic disease and has been described in greater detail on page 127. When "liver palms" have spread to involve the dorsum of the distal phalanx, as they sometimes do, the fingers become clubbed. Clubbing in this instance develops probably as a consequence of an increase in the blood supply to the fingertip, a pathophysiologic requisite for the drumstick deformity to occur.

Many cirrhotic patients are anemic and the pallid appearance related to hypochromia is visible in the hands of such individuals. If jaundice is a concomitant source of pigmentary effect, the characteristic sallow color seems even more pronounced in the presence of anemia. The fingernails in cirrhosis are occasionally white, opaque, and have what has been described as a "ground-glass" appearance. In contrast to the pallor of the nail bed due to anemia, the white nails of cirrhosis will not change color appreciably when blood is squeezed into the tip of the finger. This is due to the presence of an overgrowth of connective tissue which occurs between the nail plate and the bone, whereby the amount of blood available to the capillary plexus is reduced.

Arterial spiders are quite commonly found on the dorsum of the hand, and their presence correlates well with the degree of palmar

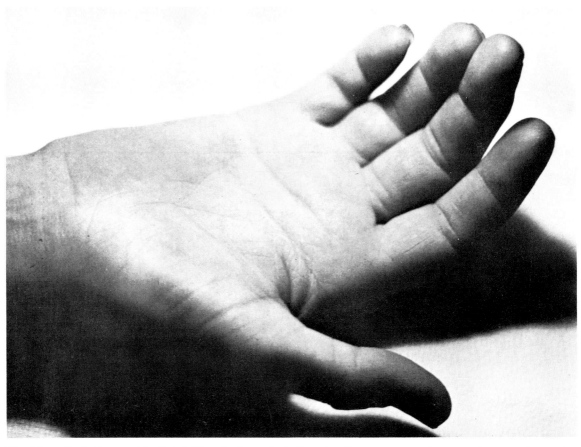

Fig. 90.   Alcoholic neuritis. Painful hand of an alcoholic who demonstrates palmar erythema and atrophy of the intrinsic musculature.

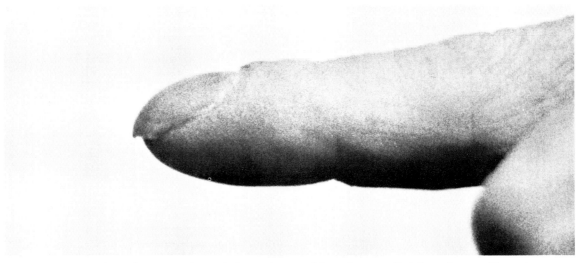

Fig. 91.   Laennec's cirrhosis. Cowling of the nail, resembling the so-called "watch-crystal" configuration.

erythema. White nails, convex nails, clubbing of the fingers, liver palms and arterial spiders are all associated with hyperestrogenism. The failure of detoxification of hormones by the damaged liver allows for the accumulation of abnormal amounts of estrogen, and is responsible for the aforementioned developments in the hand as well as the more general symptoms and signs of alopecia, gynecomastia and relative impotence.

Ecchymoses are seen in many cirrhotic patients owing to defects in the prothrombin complex and in part are due to an associated nutritional deficiency in the vessel walls, particularly on the dorsum of the hand where the vasculature is most vulnerable to trauma. Other effects of nutritional inadequacy are present in the nails where transverse grooves (Beau's lines) or ridges occur, and irregularities in the structure of the nail plate produce many types of deformity.

The tremendously elevated levels of serum lipids in biliary cirrhosis are usually associated with xanthomas in the skin. Often these occur in the creases of the palm and fingers. Xanthomas appear either as yellow or tan ribbons of fat cells, or in the tuberous form which are larger fleshy nodules that are sometimes of sufficiently great size to impair normal mechanical operation of the hand (see page 120).

Many alcoholics will become afflicted with peripheral neuritis and it is not uncommon that the hands of these individuals will be involved in such a process. As a result of the pain of neuritis and the generalized nutritional disorder, the muscles of the hand are sometimes tender and atrophic with a diminished muscle mass.

Hypertrophy of the palmar fascia occurs significantly more often in persons with hepatic cirrhosis than in the general population. The process begins and develops in the same manner as, and is indistinguishable from, Dupuytren's contracture seen in non-cirrhotics. As the dense fibrous extensions of the palmar aponeurosis become thicker and shorter, the digits are drawn toward the palm in the same order of frequency as is observed in other forms of this disorder; that is, the fourth finger is most often involved, followed in decreasing order of frequency by the fifth, the third and the index finger. Although I have no statistical confirmation of the impression, it seems that Dupuytren's contracture is observed in combination with palmar erythema among non-cirrhotics in a greater percentage than could be explained on chance findings alone.

6 *Miscellaneous* DISORDERS INVOLVING THE HAND

PALMAR ERYTHEMA

The term "liver palms," more correctly called "palmar erythema," has been applied to the reddened skin in the hands of individuals who have liver disease. Scholarly and meticulous observation of this phenomenon by Bean, Walshe and Becker and others over the past generation has extended our understanding of its relationship with other pathologic and physiologic entities beyond cirrhosis.

Palmar erythema refers to a constant mottled redness in the skin which usually begins as a sharply outlined patch in the heel of the hand. As it advances and becomes more extensive it involves progressively the ulnar edge of the palm and the fleshy limits of the hypothenar muscle pad. With further extension it spreads around the heel of the hand to include the thenar area and the cushions in the palm overlying the metacarpal heads. Occasionally, it progresses to the tips of the fingers and even colors the extensor surfaces of the distal phalanx at the base of the nails. Usually, at this stage of involvement, clubbing of the fingers occurs since the necessary vascular criteria are thereby fulfilled for the development of clubbing. More often, however, palmar erythema is confined to the parts of the hand which would ordinarily come in contact with a surface, such as in making a palm print.

An increase in blood flow and in skin temperature in the erythematous areas has been reported. The number of capillaries is also increased in the affected areas and capillary pulsations are sometimes visible. Silverstein suggests the presence of spontaneous arteriovenous shunts in the affected tissues. Sufficient evidence exists to relate liver palms with estrogenic disorders. The damaged liver is unable to neutralize circulating estrogen and the resultant hyperestrogenism is responsible for numerous gonadal and dermal stigmata. In the male cirrhotics the effects of high levels of female hormones cause gynecomastia, and pectoral, axillary and, sometimes, pubic alopecia, and testicular atrophy. Spider angiomata are associated with elevated estrogen levels and with palmar erythema; the two conditions are common in hepatic disease and in pregnancy. Sixty-two per cent of white pregnant women and 35 per cent of pregnant Negresses examined by Bean had palmar erythema and most of them had vascular spiders also. Shortly after parturition the erythema faded and disappeared and it was possible to cause it to reappear to a lesser degree by the administration of estradiol.

The same redness of the palms occurs in other conditions such as rheumatoid arthritis, mitral insufficiency, vitamin deficiencies and diabetes mellitus. A painful type of palmar erythema attended by vague paresthesias has been described in dry beri-beri. A form of palmar erythema has been found in patients who demonstrated the shoulder-hand syndrome following myocardial infarction.

Certain patients with pulmonary tuberculosis will have color changes in their hands. Acroerythrosis is a diffuse homogeneous redness which is seen in the fingers and palms and differs in appearance from the usual blotchy more localized palmar erythema seen in other tuberculous individuals.

In some patients with palmar erythema there is a similar redness present on the sole of the foot.

About 3 to 5 per cent of normal people have palmar erythema and attempts to ascribe an underlying pathologic cause for its appearance in these individuals have been unsuccessful.

EDEMA OF THE HAND

Edema of the tissues occurs in a wide variety of pathologic conditions and is usually generalized throughout the body except when gravitational factors cause it to settle into dependent parts. Major etiologic categories of generalized edema are cardiac, renal, hepatic, metabolic, and nutritional. When edema is limited to a fairly well-localized area such as one extremity or a part of a limb, the underlying mechanism is usually vascular or lymphatic obstruction, or inflammation. Occasionally, tissue fluid will accumulate on one side of the body, collecting in the upper and lower extremity of the same side due to the position assumed by the patient in recumbency, although the underlying condition may be basically a generalized edema.

Discussion here is concerned with localized edema of the hand and its possible causes. Inflammatory factors are perhaps most frequently encountered such as cellulitis, soft tissue abscesses, phlebitis, or thrombosis.

Circumscribed areas of reddened, non-tender edema are more likely due to arteriolar dilatation in areas of edema where tenderness is a feature and an increase in local temperature is suggestive of an inflammatory cause. Cyanotic edema is more usually due to venous outflow obstruction. Impediment to venous or lymphatic drainage at any point proximal to the edema is often related to the presence of an obstructing mass situated in the axilla, the cervical triangle, or in the upper or anterior mediastinum. When the findings are bilateral, edema, distention and tortuosity of the superficial veins of the face, neck, upper extremities and anterior chest wall indicate obstruction of the superior vena cava., The superior vena caval syndrome refers to interference with venous return to the right atrium from the upper part of the body and frequently is due to the presence of a neoplasm in the superior thoracic outlet, the mediastinum, or at the pulmonary apex. An aneurysm of the ascending or transverse arches of the aorta may exert sufficient pressure on the superior vena cava to produce edema in the arms. When compression is limited to only one innominate or subclavian vein, the edema is unilateral. Venous distention occurs in the tributaries to the vena cava and a cyanotic plethora is a striking finding in the same areas. The clinical signs of the superior vena caval syndrome are sharply accentuated by the recumbent position and are eased somewhat by an upright or sitting posture. The hand becomes dusky and swollen, and the dark dilated veins on the dorsum will not empty as readily when the hands are elevated above the patient's head due to an increased venous pressure.

A rough estimation of venous pressure has valid clinical application in a well-known simple bedside procedure. This method consists in raising the individual's hand slowly above his head and measuring the height necessary to empty the veins on the dorsum of the hand. Venous emptying should begin when the hand is at the level of the atrium, but the point at which it occurs is significantly higher in congestive heart failure, the superior vena caval syndrome, and in any other condition associated with elevated venous pressure.

Occasionally, edema of one or both arms occurs in nephrosis and in certain instances of nephritis. In the elderly, but otherwise normal individual, and more often in the patient with varying degrees of

Fig. 92. Lymphedema. Edematous left arm and hand secondary to the effects of radical amputation of the breast (for carcinoma) and consequent removal of axillary lymphatic structures.

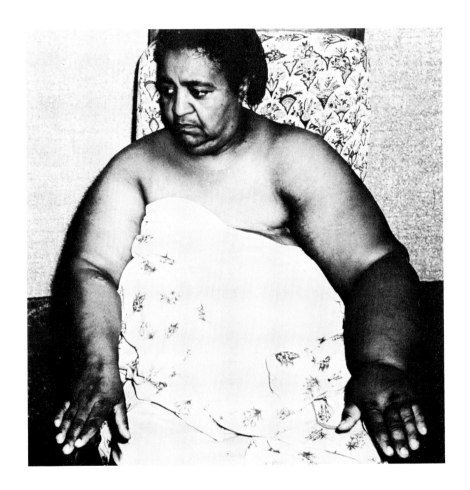

congestive heart failure, the position in bed during sleep may account for edema formation in one arm and the leg on the same side, the dependent side collecting detectable amounts of fluid overnight as an effect of gravity. Patients with malnutrition and hypoproteinemia, although usually showing generalized edema, may demonstrate localized edema in the upper extremities and face.

Among the other causes for edema of the hand are Raynaud's disease, myositis, cervical rib, tumor of the hand, Hodgkin's disease (axillary lymphadenomegaly), mediastinitis, trichiniasis, and syringomyelia ("the succulent hand of Marinesco"). Hemiplegia following a cerebrovascular accident frequently causes edema in the paralyzed hand as also is manifest in many instances in which there is damage to the motor function of the hand.

Following radical mastectomy, which includes excision of axillary lymphatic structures, a troublesome lymphedema of the upper extremity and hand on the operated side frequently rises to a symptomatic level.

Carcinoma of the breast with metastasis to the regional lymph nodes or aneurysm of the axillary artery may cause pressure on the neighboring veins and be responsible for edema formation in the hands. Axillary abscess or compression from a cluster of enlarged lymph nodes in the axilla, fairly commonplace in Hodgkin's disease or leukemia, can produce vascular obstruction sufficient to cause swelling distal to it.

SENILE CHANGES IN THE HAND

Although advancing age cannot be considered as a disease state, its effects are unquestionably systemic and a voluminous bibliography is accumulating which documents in a scientific way the physiologic changes thus produced.

The hand participates in the alterations of senescence in an important way. One of the earliest effects of aging is the loss of manual dexterity. Surprising as it may seem, it has been estimated that manual workers first begin to lose dexterity at about age 30 and the professional man first manifests the same loss at about 35 years of age.

Contrasting the aged hand with that of a child, the major anatomic differences are to be noted in the lesser amount of subcutaneous fat in the latter years of life. As elastic tissue is diminished generally throughout the body, the "expression" of the hand is altered as age advances. The older hand is usually held more quietly, and if disease states are excluded, such as tremors and other neuro-

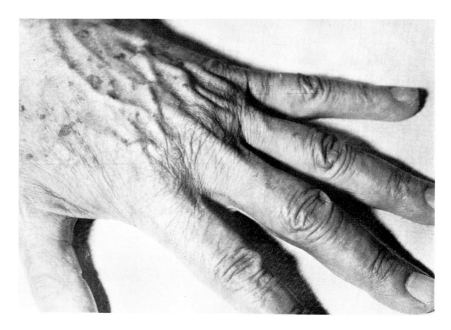

Fig. 93. Senile keratoses. Flat, slightly roughened, dirty-brown spots ("old-age spots") occur frequently on the dorsum of the hand as a mark of aging.

Fig. 94 A & B. Ischemic contracture. Cool, dry, stiff hand; fifth finger contracted and ankylosed in partial flexion, the result of ischemia caused by immobilization in a tight plaster cast for fracture of the wrist.

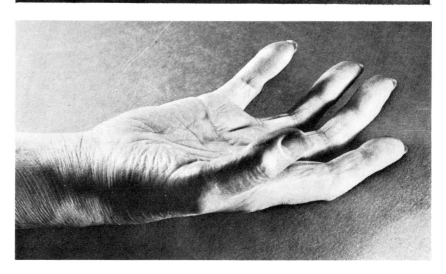

muscular disorders, there are fewer purposeless movements of the hand in the elderly. The skin is dryer, thinner, and much less resilient, and becomes whiter as it loses translucency, and wrinkled as a result of changes in skin tone. Support for the veins is lessened by the scantier subcutaneous fat layer, so that veins are more prominent, appear to be larger, are more tortuous and friable. Through the same mechanism of diminished adipose support, vessels and skin are more easily injured. Ecchymoses frequently occur and spread more readily through the looser areolar subcutaneous tissues.

Purpuric spots (senile purpura) are observed frequently in the elderly and may well be the most common of all the effects of aging to be noted in the hand. Purpura in senescence reflects not only the results of a decline in the structural support to the vein but is associated with changes in the wall of the vein itself. Certain hepatic effects of advanced age, such as deficiency in the formation of various components of the prothrombin complex, have been incriminated in the causation of senile purpura.

Other cutaneous effects are frequent such as the development of senile keratoses, "old age spots," or pigmentations and epidermoid carcinomas. Dermal epithelial cancer is encountered more often in the "weather-worn" hand and is particularly disposed to occur in the ruddy-complexioned, freckled type of individual who has demonstrated throughout his lifetime a resistance to tanning upon exposure to sunlight.

Certain other trophic changes are age-linked, such as Heberden's nodes, which are inherited as a mendelian dominant characteristic in women and as a recessive trait among men (see page 20). It is doubtful that these nodes represent a wear-and-tear phenomenon per se, since they are found just as often in individuals who have no occupational reason for their presence. An associated overpull of digital tendons causes deviation or angulation from the straight line of the terminal phalanx of the finger either laterally or medially.

Compared with a younger person, contraction deformities occur more readily in the hand of an aged patient as a serious sequela to prolonged fixation in plaster for the treatment of fractures about the elbow or wrist.

In advanced years, arterial circulation in the extremities has considerably narrower reserves so that lesser circulatory impediments from trauma or occlusive pressures are required to produce anoxic effect which might not be of sufficient magnitude to affect a younger individual.

Reflex neuromuscular dystrophic effects such as the "shoulder-hand syndrome" are more prevalent in middle life and later, as phenomena related to various remote mechanical factors (see

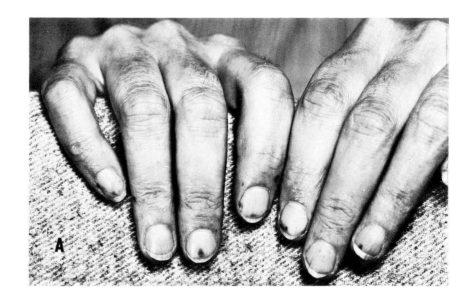

Fig. 95 A & B. Hereditary hemorrhagic telangiectasia. Hemorrhagic spots under the nails and in the skin of the fingers associated with epistaxis and dilatation of capillaries and venules in the skin and mucous membranes throughout the body. Lesions may produce bleeding from the gastrointestinal, respiratory and genitourinary tract. The tourniquet test and the various components of blood are normal. (Courtesy of W. B. Bean.)

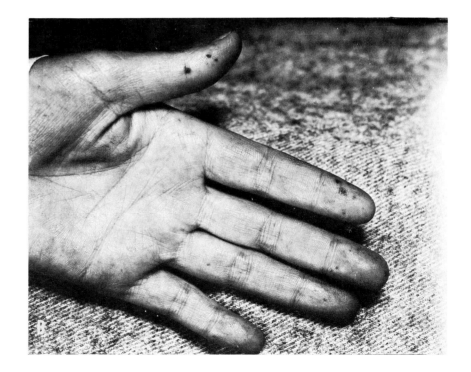

"Shoulder-Hand Syndrome"). Calcific tendonitis at the shoulder, post-myocardial infarctional sclerodactylia, neoplasm at the superior thoracic outlet, or in the mediastinum, and several other causative mechanisms for the shoulder-hand syndrome are mentioned elsewhere in this text.

The carpal tunnel syndrome is another local manifestation of a number of mechanical and inflammatory conditions which cause median nerve compression under the ligaments at the wrist. Commonest causes for the painful symptoms (as outlined on page 45) are rheumatoid arthritis, malunited fractures, and tenosynovitis. Although the carpal tunnel syndrome is most often seen in the menopausal woman, there appears to be a definite age incidence with a greater frequency as age advances.

HEREDITARY HEMORRHAGIC TELANGIECTASIA (Osler's Disease; Rendu-Osler-Weber Disease)

The diagnosis of hereditary hemorrhagic telangiectasia should be considered by the physician faced with the problem of diagnosis in a child or young adult who has recurrent epistaxis, particularly when there exists a history of similar bleeding episodes in other members of the family. A study of the coagulogram in these individuals is completely unrewarding in a positive way, since coagulation defects are lacking. Important diagnostic clues are provided by the presence of small punctate telangiectatic lesions that are associated with the disease.

Like most heritable diseases, this condition is usually first encountered in the young patient in whom its onset is generally heralded by a bleeding tendency, often in the form of brisk nosebleeds.

The classic lesions are spidery or punctiform telangiectases which are flat or slightly depressed, red or purple spots clearly demarcated from the surrounding skin or mucous membranes. Pressure causes the lesions to fade completely except only rarely, when blanching may be somewhat short of complete. Occasionally a ring of white dry scales surrounds the lesions, especially those which are found on the fingers. Red or dark mahogany blotches may be seen under the nail plate. Such localized areas of inadequate, fragile, vascular structures represent the cardinal pathologic sign of this clinical disorder.

An associated pulmonary arteriovenous fistula should be searched for when hemorrhagic telangiectasia is discovered in the skin or mucous membrane.

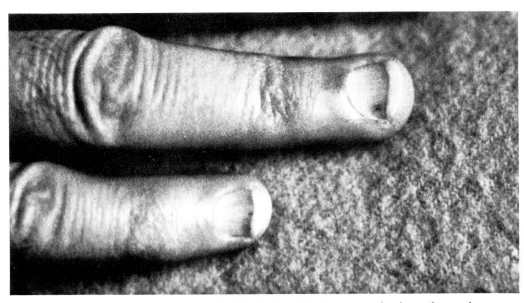

Fig. 96. Hemorrhagic "fringe." At distal end of nail bed, a type of splinter hemorrhage seen in blood dyscrasias accompanied by bleeding tendencies. This patient had hypofibrinogenemia secondary to widespread carcinomatosis. Primary tumor in pancreas.

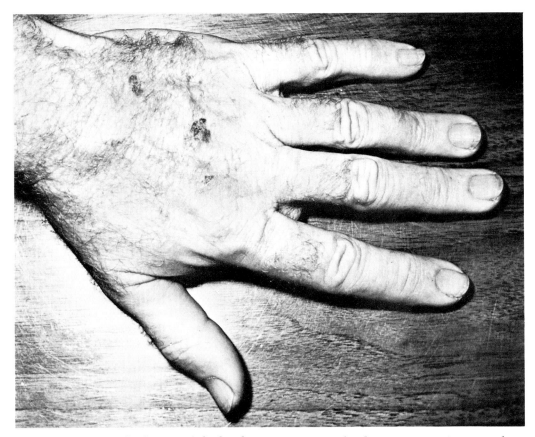

Fig. 97. Purpura. The dorsum of the hand is a common site for demonstration of purpura from any cause.

HEMATOLOGIC DISEASES

ANEMIA

The normal color of flesh derives from a number of physical factors, one of which is the concentration of hemoglobin and other pigments visible through the stratum corneum. Color values vary when circulatory dynamics increase or diminish the delivery of these pigments to the skin surface. The trained eye is capable of detecting variations from the normal and may gather helpful clinical diagnostic information by adding it to other available parameters.

Pallor of the skin and mucous membranes has long been associated with anemic states. The presence of other pigments, and circulatory or dermal effects, may modify the interpretations possible. In the white race the color of the palmar creases supplies more valid information than do other parts of the hand including the nail base in the detection of anemia. The palmar creases are normally some shade of pink but become pale or silvery white when the hemoglobin concentration falls to abnormal levels. Wintrobe correlates the appearance of this color change to a critical hemoglobin level at approximately 7 grams per 100 ml. of blood.

In addition to palmar pallor, certain trophic changes are noted frequently as effects of nutritional deficit consequent to anemia. Such nutritional changes are likely to affect nail and nail bed structures with the formation of bizarre shapes such as spoon nails, crinkling of the nail surfaces or edges of the nails, abnormal separations from the nail bed, Mee's lines, Beau's lines, and vertical ridging of the nail plate.

PURPURA

Most diseases which have purpuric manifestations will be attended by evidence of the disorder in the hand at one time or another. This is accounted for by the frequency with which minor traumas occur to the relatively vulnerable dorsum of the hand, and the superficial position of numerous vessels backed up by the rigid metacarpal bones. In the senile hand, supporting soft tissue is in shorter supply than in the juvenile hand, and the vessels are more tortuous, fragile, and frequently more distended. Senile purpura, a common entity in the elderly, shows a definite predilection for occurrence in the skin of the back of the hand. Petechial hemorrhages, however, are more frequently situated in the palm and on the pads of the fingers.

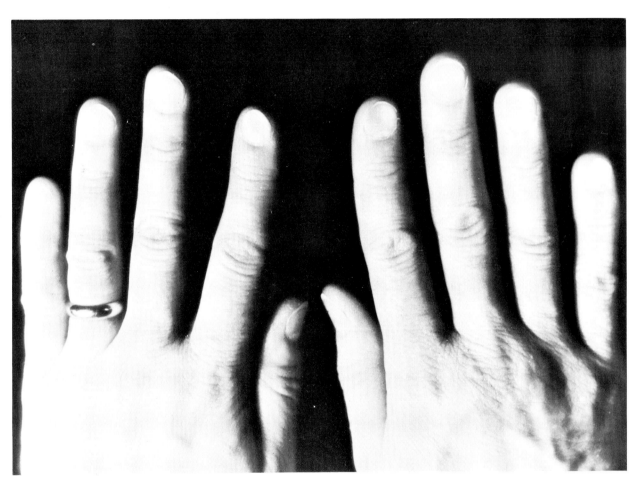

Fig. 98. Plummer-Vinson syndrome. Hands of a patient with Plummer-Vinson syndrome, associated with dysphagia and anemia. Concave nails are most prominently demonstrated in the index and middle fingers.

Generalized purpuric rashes may be severe enough in certain instances to run along all of the major and secondary creases in the palm and fingers, producing a blue to violet network of pigmentation over the entire hand.

PLUMMER-VINSON SYNDROME

Usually the descriptive term "spoon nails" (koilonychia) is immediately linked with a systemic disorder, the Plummer-Vinson syndrome. Several other clinical entities, however, may demonstrate the same type of concave nail plate. For example, spoon nails are seen in hypothyroidism and in simple hypochromic anemias. Acromegaly, polycythemia, secondary syphilis, nutritional deficiencies, and certain circulatory disorders such as coronary sclerosis may also produce spoon-nail deformity. Inadequate circulation to the digits from any mechanism may allow for the development of spoon nails.

The identification of the Plummer-Vinson syndrome is possible by observation of several characteristic features which classically occur in this interesting entity, usually suggested by a dysmenorrheic, anemic, dysphagic female. The patient afflicted with this syndrome usually demonstrates a characteristically thin and pallid skin, poor dentition, and exhibits a predisposition to develop peptic ulceration or malignant lesions of the upper gastrointestinal tract.

As part of the clinical picture of the Plummer-Vinson syndrome, ectodermal dysplasia is considered to be responsible for changes in the nail plates. The surfaces of the nails become concave, spooned, or flattened. The phenomenon is seen initially and most prominently in the thumb and first three fingers. With advancement of the defect, all the fingernails may be involved.

SICKLE-CELL ANEMIA

A form of chronic hereditary hemolytic anemia is found in the Negro and is characterized by the presence of abnormal types of hemoglobin. Individuals with the pure form of the disease (homozygous S-S hemoglobin) are frequently of an asthenic bodily habitus (see Fig. 47). They usually have a short trunk and long slender entremities. Their hips and shoulders are narrow and they are frequently underweight. The palms of the hands and the mucous membranes and sclerae are greenish-yellow and spider fingers (arachnodactyly) are common.

The erythrocytes are usually sickle-shaped or oat-shaped, a phenomenon which is enhanced under conditions of reduced oxygenation. Clinically, there are rheumatoid manifestations including swell-

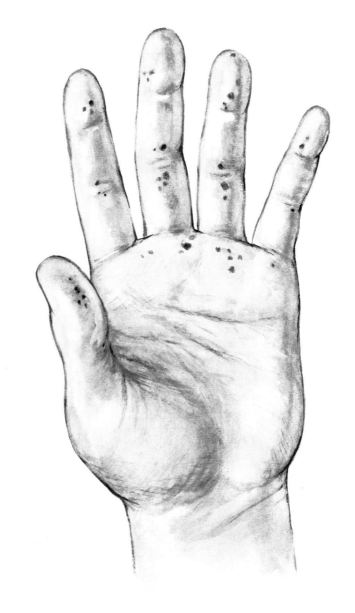

Fig. 99. Peutz-Jegher syndrome. Pigmented spots on the hand associated with intestinal polyposis in the Peutz-Jegher syndrome. Usually the same type of melanin deposits is present in the oral mucosa and around the lips and nostrils.

ing and redness of the joints which resemble, in some instances, the manifestations of an acute arthritis. Acute attacks of abdominal pain occur in episodes and closely mimic acute surgical conditions. A leukocytosis, tenderness in the abdomen, and fever up to 103° F. may add to the diagnostic difficulties.

The long slender asthenic hands and feet and spidery fingers are commonly observed in sickle-cell anemia. Wintrobe reports an instance of hypoplasia of the terminal phalanx of one of the fingers in a patient with sickle-cell disease.

The observation of the characteristic appearance of the hand may be helpful in the differential diagnosis of patients with evidence of hemolytic anemia and what appears to be an acute abdominal emergency.

PEUTZ-JEGHER SYNDROME

Polyposis of the intestines is an hereditary disease which is characterized by the presence of multiple varisized polyps which are located predominantly in the mucosa of the small bowel, and pigmented spots in the skin and mucous membranes. A frequent site of these black or dark brown spots is around the mouth, especially the lower lip, and to a lesser extent around the nostrils, eyelids, hands, and feet. They tend to fade as age progresses.

The intestinal polyps have a tendency to bleed or cause intussusception but only rarely do they become malignant. Pallor, due to the anemia produced by hemorrhages from the polyps, accentuates the appearance of melanin deposits in the skin. The deposits are oval or irregularly round and are clearly demarcated from the normal skin. They are usually distributed in the hands over the palmar aspects of the fingers.

Several interesting variations of this syndrome have been reported, one of which combines intestinal hemangiomas with similar pigmentation in and around the mouth and hands. Small, red, non-blanching, flame-shaped hemangiomas are found in the palm and sole in addition to the black to dark brown macules on the dorsum of the hand.

TUBEROUS SCLEROSIS

Tuberous sclerosis is one of the neurodermatoses and carries the descriptive adjective *tuberous* which refers to the potato-like appearance of the damaged cerebral cortex. This disease is characterized by epileptic seizures, mental deficiencies, acneform skin disorders, and intracranial calcifications. Dystrophic effects are noted in the fingernails which are frequently grooved longitudinally and become distorted and split by the presence of slowly growing subungual fibromas. Supernumerary digits and syndactylism are encountered quite often in patients with tuberous sclerosis. A large variety and distribution of neoplasms are encountered throughout the body including hypernephromas and rhabdomyomas of the heart.

MAFFUCCI'S SYNDROME

A rare inborn error in the genesis of cartilage and bone has the eponymic designation of Maffucci's syndrome. It is responsible for a dramatic clinical misadventure in bodily configuration and proportion. A common denominator from a pathologic standpoint is the association of hemangioma, dyschondroplasia, and occasionally phlebectasia. The usual onset occurs with the formation of a small nodule on a finger or a toe. This appears as a soft, non-tender, purplish hemangioma which is surrounded by small dilated venules and which progresses ultimately to the formation of an endochondroma. Such swellings progress in an irregular fashion until the most incredibly grotesque dyssymmetries of the human form are produced. Occasionally, there is a curious mottling of the palms, the trunk, and upper extremities. A high incidence of malignant degeneration is observed in cartilaginous structures and sarcomatous changes occur often in the blood vessels as terminal events. There is often noted a striking difference in the comparative size of the extremities in which one hand may be smaller or asymmetric enlargements occur. Sometimes one or more fingers may be irregularly misshaped.

LAURENCE-MOON-BIEDL SYNDROME

This syndrome embraces a constellation of congenital abnormalities which includes obesity, mental deficiency, retinitis pigmentosa, and hypogenitalism. Like so many other developmental disorders it is frequently associated with polydactylism and syndactylism. There are very few instances of dysgerminisms in which some abnormality in the form or functional development of the hand is not a concomitant event.

MISCELLANEOUS DISORDERS **142**

HAND-BITING

In certain mentally defective individuals, self-mutilation may occur in the form of hand-biting. Such a neurotic impulse seems to arise most frequently from strong feelings of resentment, frustration, or anger. Similar abnormal behavior is demonstrated in monkeys when they become excited or enraged. Under such a circumstance they have been observed to sit down and bite their feet furiously. Human beings more often find the hand or forearm more accessible for such a practice.

All gradations of self-inflicted damage to the bitten parts are possible. Nail-biting (onychophagia), cuticle-chewing or -tearing, callus-picking, and the like, are more commonly encountered in lower order neuroses which ordinarily have a sharply diminished incidence at puberty. Persistence of the habit into the adult years usually is indicative of a mild personality disorder stemming from tension, frustration, and attitudes of insecurity. Detrimental effects appear to be limited to cosmetic import.

Another, higher order variant of the practice of self-biting is knuckle- and thumb-biting in children and some immature, neurotic adults. Such persons repeatedly attack the same general area of the hand or digit with vigorous chewing, usually stopping just short of what would be painful to them. They will only very seldom break through the skin with their teeth. The severity of the habit and its consequences are motivated by the individual's characteristic response to situations of stressful meditation or periods of excitement or nervous tension. The habit is often acquired by the susceptible subject through mimicry of parents, associates, or fellow inmates. Deeper psychologic mechanisms of suppressed anger, revenge, or resentment are possible underlying causes for hand-biting.

About 2 per cent of feeble-minded inmates of a state institution are hand-biters. Repeated trauma from sucking and chewing along the radial and dorsal surfaces of the lower arm and hand produces characteristic and permanent disfigurement of the skin. Pigmented, indurated, oval or elliptical marks result from such practices. Hyperemia induced by sucking, and the excessive moisture due to saliva on the involved skin surface, often causes an overgrowth of long, luxuriant hair which follows the oval outline of the area included in the bite.

Figs. 100-107 (pages 144-147). Hand-biting in psychotics. Several examples of effects of self-biting in the hands of mentally defective subjects. Habitual sucking on the dorsum of the hand causes hyperemia and hypertrichosis localized to the same area. (Courtesy of Thos. Butterworth, Pa. Medical Journal.)

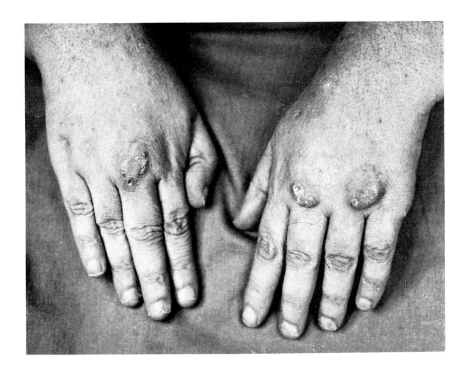

Fig. 100

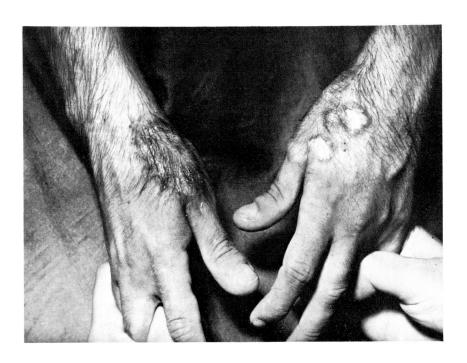

Fig. 101

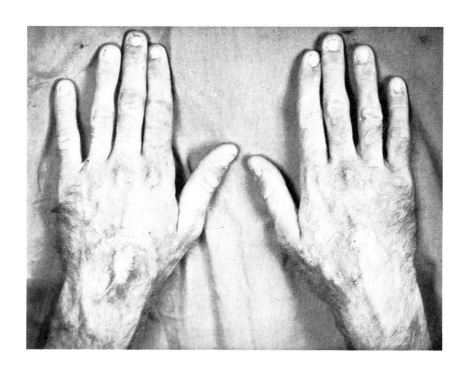

Fig. 102

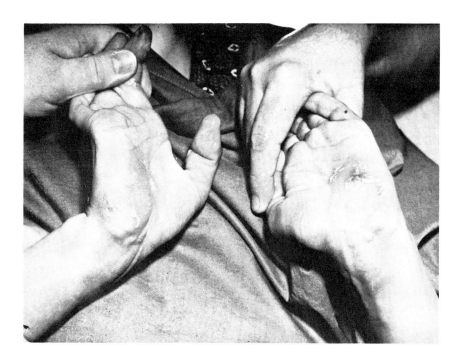

Fig. 103

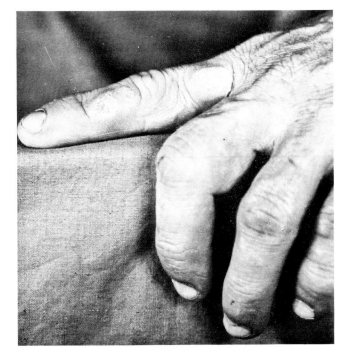

Fig. 104

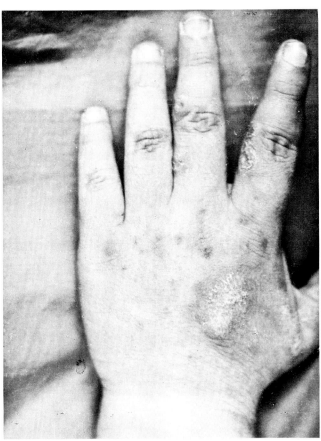

Fig. 105

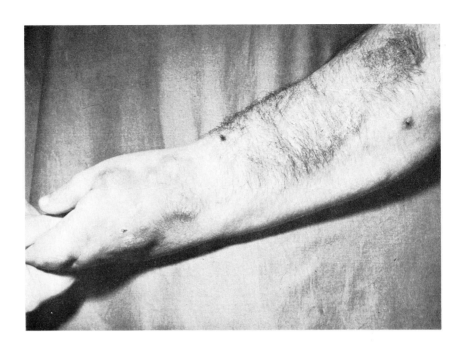

Fig. 106

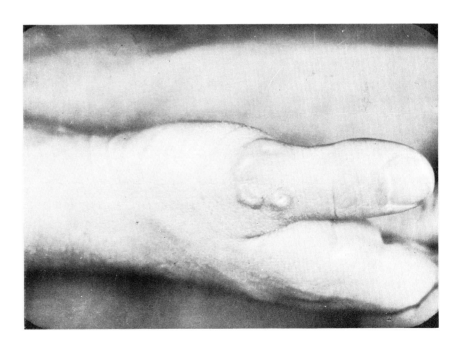

Fig. 107

OCCUPATIONAL EFFECTS IN THE HAND

"The hand of little employment hath the daintier sense."
—*Wm. Shakespeare, Hamlet, V. 1*

In a general way, characteristic physical signs can be observed in the hand as a result of adaptation in normal individuals to the manner of the use of the hand in work or play. Repeated pressures or friction on particular parts of the hand cause the formation of protective calluses in appropriate locations. The effects of wear may be evident in one area of the hand or another, and the exceptional development of all or part of the intrinsic musculature follows the simple laws of hypertrophy through usage. The reverse is also true—the inactive hand is innocent of the well-known signs of wear and tear. Thus, a simple inspection of the hand, observing the stains, scars, and calluses, is sufficient to allow for an immediate evaluation of some points of varying importance which add to the examiner's knowledge of his patient. Occasionally, such knowledge has medicolegal value, and has been helpful in the identification of an unconscious patient whose hands suggested his occupation by the presence of telltale stains or marks. Although automation and the use of appropriate apparel and protective devices have in some considerable measure thwarted the effects of friction and other external irritants on the hands, there still remains many types of manual labor which inflict recognizable signs of wear on the hands.

The initial hyperemic response of soft tissue to repeated friction and pressure leads progressively to local edema, possibly with blister formation, and ultimately to the development of callus. The advantage thus gained permits further exposure to similar traumatic experience with some degree of protective immunity to its harmful effects. The sheets of keratin and callus thrown up against the ravages of painful wear thus represent a successful tissue adaptation. Fortunately they are acquired quite readily, but will fade and disappear soon after the cause is no longer active. Rarely an individual is unable to form callus, such as the patient with epidermolysis bullosa. In such patients, slight friction will produce painful blisters which are not followed by callus formation. These persons are therefore not suited for employment in occupations which require hard use of the hands.

The thick-skinned hand of the laborer is easily distinguished from the soft, finely textured hand of the office worker, but it must be remembered that hobbies or sports may inflict the marks of the manual laborer upon the white-collar worker.

Ronchese has written extensively upon the subject of "occupational marks" and has compiled an impressive array of external

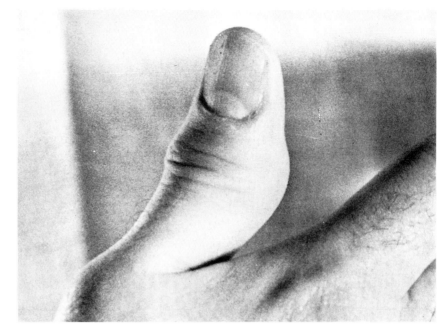

Fig. 108. Bowler's thumb. Thickened thumb joint which developed as a result of many years of bowling.

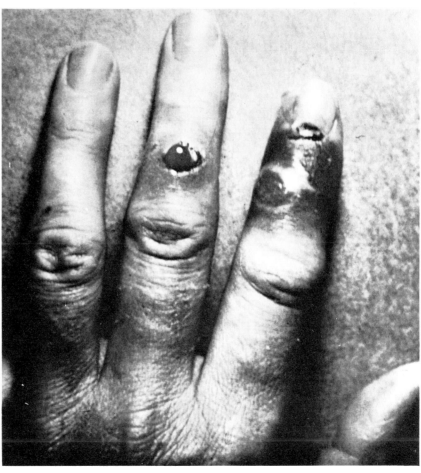

Fig. 109. Orf. Pyogenic lesions contracted by sheep-handlers.

signs acquired in persons exposed to various occupational environments. For the most complete description of these effects the reader is referred to Ronchese's excellent text.

Some of the visible effects of work are due to stains, pigments, or tattoos. The draftsman or bookkeeper may exhibit blue-black penpoint marks on the dorsum of his hand or in the inter-digital webbing where inadvertent tattooing is frequent. The laboratory technician's fingers may be stained yellow or brown from handling acids. Picklers and hatters show yellow stains on the skin of the hand and textile or leather workers who are exposed to oxalic acid sometimes develop a blue discoloration of the nails. The photographic finisher usually has brown, silver-stained fingertips. Polishers of various types have shiny, smooth, stained skin and worn nails. House painters not only exhibit the effects of contact with pigment under the fingernails, and a skin which is dried and defatted from the effects of turpentine, but may develop disabling wristdrop from lead neuropathy. Mirror manufacturers have their employees examined frequently and watched closely for evidence of radial nerve weakness, a potential hazard to workers engaged in the silvering process. The silversmith may absorb sufficient particles to color the skin of his hands a slate-blue gray. Blueness of the nail beds in argyria does not blanch out with pressure, in contrast with the cyanotic fingertip. Grinders may demonstrate a speckled tattoo due to flying bits of metal which become embedded in the skin on the dorsum of their hands.

Chemical handlers and workers in refineries are especially prone to develop skin rashes of a variety of kinds, chiefly acneform or eczematous, due to contact with chemical or thermal irritants. No effort will be made to list the multitude of possible offending chemical agents used in industry, and, to be sure, the attempt would commit unnecessary duplication. Full accounts are available in suitable reference volumes.

Although it may have limited value as a diagnostic clue it is often of interest to study the location of callus in the hands of the patient (or note its absence) and to attempt, when possible, to assign its proper significance. Handles of shovels and steering wheels of automobiles may cause a transverse linear callus in the palm near the base of the fingers. Brief-case or sample-case carriers may demonstrate a thickening of the skin in the same place as do shovelers. Rakers and sweepers build callus in the webbing between the thumb and index finger. The determined housewife develops a circular or linear ridge in the palmar skin from her grip on the electric iron.

Many bakers develop a characteristic callus on the heel of the hand induced by handling baking trays, hot from the ovens. A

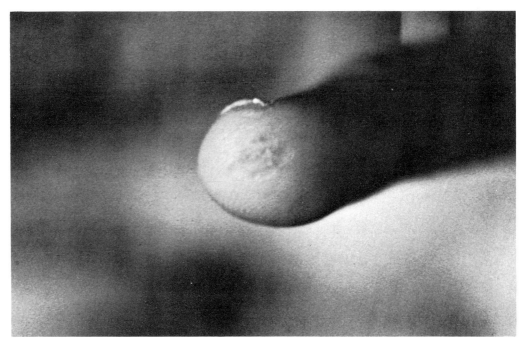

Fig. 110. Cellist's callus. Showing location of callus on the tip of the fifth finger on the left hand of a cello player.

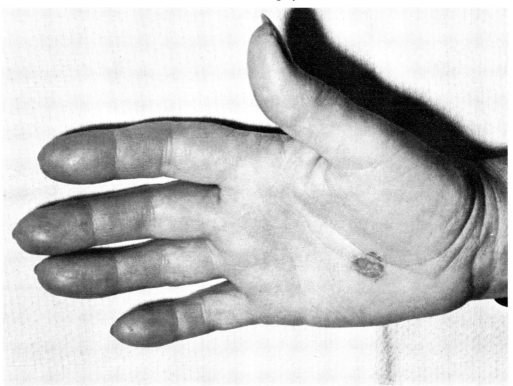

Fig. 111. Gardener's callus. Common location for callus in the hobbyist gardener due to pressure from the handle of a trowel.

MISCELLANEOUS DISORDERS

mycotic infection caused by a yeast-like organism occurs occasionally in the web between the middle and third finger among kitchen workers or bakers. The flesh in this area becomes soggy, pale and ulcerated and closely resembles the lesion seen in epidermophytosis of the foot.

The oft-maligned butcher's thumb may show a telltale sign in the outside corner of the nail which may be shaved on the angle. "Butcher's pemphigus" is a bullous lesion of far less severity than its name implies, which usually appears within 48 hours after inoculation of a septic wound on the hand. Cattle handlers or slaughterhouse workers exposed to infected beef or pork may develop a papulo-pustular lesion of the hand which has the general appearance of a contact dermatitis. Pinpoint papules develop within a few hours of inoculation and eventually become pustular. Such a lesion is due to infection with the Brucella organism.

"Milker's nodules" are hemispherical, bean-sized, tender, red nodules which form on the dorsum of the thumb and index finger of dairy workers. The nodule may be covered with a red, brown or brick-colored dark crust or may be umbilicated. Tenderness and swelling of the finger and elbow joints may follow the digital lesions. At one time these nodules were thought to be due to a foreign body reaction around a cow's hair which had penetrated the skin of the milker's hand. It is now well-established that the etiologic agent is a virus (pox virus).

The tip of the cellist's fifth finger and all of the fingertips (left) of the violinist exhibit thin, rough calluses. The strength and muscular control of the hands required of the pianist is not fully appreciated by those who are unfamiliar with the instrument. Rigorous exercise and exceptional energy expenditures over prolonged periods result in a degree of muscular development in the hands of the accomplished pianist. This is contrary to the usual impression of the long, slender, delicate hands pictured by the unobserving. Glass blowers and persons who play wind instruments may develop an occupational disease of the lungs, a form of bullous emphysema. Beaking of the nails or clubbing of the fingertips may occur as a later consequence of that condition.

Workers exposed to sunlight, such as farmers and fishermen, demonstrate a ruggedness and leathery appearance in the skin of the hands and the classic quilted crease pattern on the back of the neck. Yellowish-brown or dirty-looking keratoses are seen frequently on the dorsum of the hands of individuals who spend long hours in the sun. Such persons exhibit a higher incidence of malignant disease in exposed skin areas than does the general populace. The hobbyist gardener, who shows a tendency to moniliasis of the nails, also may rub a circular patch of callus in the middle of the

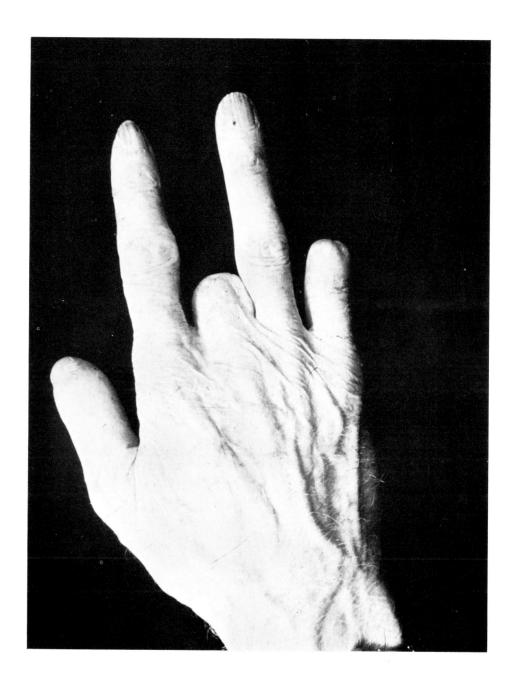

Fig. 112. Roentgen irradiation effects. The hands of a veteran radiologist show effects of unprotected, prolonged exposure to radiation. Loss of fingers or parts of digits and shaggy, hardened skin are becoming rarer owing to greater respect for the destructive action of X rays and better protective apparel. (Courtesy of American Cancer Society, Inc.)

MISCELLANEOUS DISORDERS

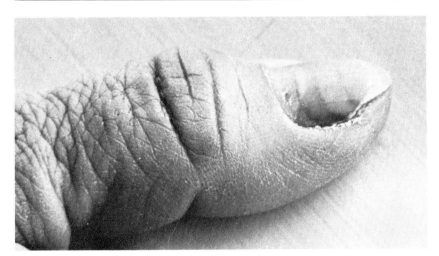

Fig. 113 A & B. Manicure marks. Colored arciform marks appearing at regularly spaced intervals in the nail which correspond to stains produced by nail lacquer.

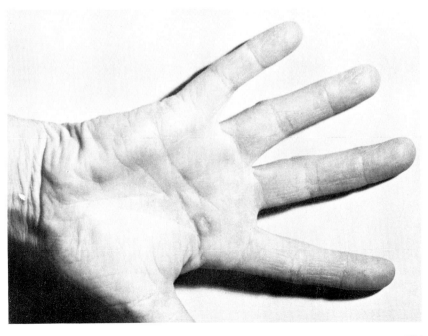

Fig. 114. Ironer's callus. Dense callus in the palm of a housewife due to an exceptionally determined grip on the iron. Callus formation may occur in the same location in persons who use a firm hold on the steering wheel of an automobile.

palm from handling a trowel. Awls and screw-drivers produce similar marks in the palm.

Many students develop "writer's nodules" which form on the radial side of the distal joint of the middle finger. Common during school years, the writer's callus disappears in later years and leaves no traces, except in a very few but obvious occupational circumstances.

Cardiologists and other physicians whose practice of percussion is a daily performance may exhibit a nodule on the dorsum of the middle phalanx of the middle finger. Occasionally, a tender ganglion may form in that location. Destruction of skin and deeper structures of the hand from prolonged unprotected exposure to roentgen radiation is a well-known mark of the veteran radiologist. Amputation of parts of digits from these effects is not uncommon among radiologists of the "old school." The nail matrix is particularly radiosensitive, which accounts for the numerous anomalies of growth and configuration in the fingernails of persons exposed to radiation effects.

Pneumatic drill operators may develop a spastic disorder of the fingers, which become white, cool and numb as a consequence of prolonged vibration of the hand-held tool.

Hairdressers who frequently handle dyes, bleaches, and other cosmetics which stain and fissure the fingertips demonstrate disfigurement of the fingernails quite regularly.

There is a well-circulated story that refers to the results of repeated injuries to the hands of professional athletes. Someone described the sensation of meeting and greeting Mr. Yogi Berra, the celebrated catcher on the New York Yankee baseball team.

"Shaking hands with Yogi is just like sticking your hand into a bowl of pretzels."

Thickened joints and bent but strong fingers of the baseball player are scars of the trade acquired by even the most expert performer and carried forever as marks of the veteran. Golfers, tennis players, and those engaged in various other sports, either for purposes of recreation or livelihood, will incur callus-formation in the hands, or effects of injuries which are more or less specific for the particular activity.

Innumerable instances of similar occupational marks of use in the hand could be set down but would duplicate other reference sources and veer somewhat off the course of my original intent. Let it be sufficient, then, for my purpose to recall what is obvious and well-known, that the elementary use of careful inspection is a valid means of acquiring information, useful or otherwise, about the patient. To the physician receptive to such easily available data, the hand offers eloquent testimony of its use as an occupational tool.

SUBSULTUS TENDINUM

A venerable physical sign, described in most old medical textbooks, but which is not mentioned in either of the current major reference works on Internal Medicine, is "subsultus tendinum" or "carphologia." The criteria of what is or is not clinically important has shifted noticeably as our latter day diagnostic armamentarium requires less of the minutiae at the bedside and a proportionately greater reliance upon the laboratory sciences.

For certain, the knowledge that spasmodic twitching of the tendons about the wrist and fingers is a phenomenon frequently associated with profound febrile states will not measurably enhance the clinician's diagnostic acumen, but I have acceded to a compulsion by including it here.

Nervous, aimless picking at the bedclothing has the same vague clinical significance and historical background. In deference to the earliest description of this sign, the following quotation is offered:

"Respecting the movement of the hands I have these observations to make: when in acute fevers, pneumonia, phrenitis, or headache, the hands are waved before the face, hunting through empty space, as if gathering bits of straw, picking the nap from the coverlet, or beating chaff from the wall—all such symptoms are bad and deadly."
—*Hippocrates, (The Book of Prognostics)*

ARSENICAL TOXICITY

The neural and dermal effects of chronic arsenical toxicity may cause striking physical changes in the hand, or in certain instances may be limited altogether to the palms and soles. Early and outstanding signs of toxicity from the ingestion of arsenic, either inadvertently or in the form of medication, are excessive sweating and sharply outlined erythema in the palm. The soles of the feet also may be involved in an identical process at the same time. Wrist drop, due to radial neuritis, and multiple paralyses are not uncommon as consequences of toxic polyneuritis caused by arsenic. Eczematoid eruptions, pruritus, and secondary infection of the palms progress to an exfoliative dermatitis which heals eventually with hyperpigmentation (arsenical melanosis).

Extensive keratoses of the palm and dorsum of the hand are outstanding characteristics of arsenical poisoning. They resemble senile keratoses or, on occasion, may assume a light-yellow, circumscribed, warty type of configuration. There is a tendency for these lesions to undergo malignant change in as many as 20 per cent of the subjects. Arsenical keratotic lesions may appear early, within a few weeks after ingestion of arsenic, or may not develop for many years after exposure. The favorite sites for their appearance are in areas where friction or calluses are present. Destruction and shedding of the nails may occur. Changes in the hand resembling scleroderma have been reported to occur as sequelae of arsenical toxicity.

Arsenic demonstrates an affinity for localization in epithelial structures and can be isolated and identified by chemical techniques in hair, skin, and nails. Light- or dark-grayish transverse bands, Mee's lines, appear in the nails at the lunula, about eight weeks after exposure to the toxic agent and gradually grow out distally. Higher concentrations of arsenic are detectable in these bands than in the remainder of the nail. Beau's lines, which are cross ridges in the nail plate, may be found in some persons having arsenical poisoning and have the same significance as do Mee's lines or leukonychia striata. An approximation of the date of ingestion of the poison is possible by measurement of the nail bands or ridges and calculating on the basis of one millimeter of nail growth for every 10 days.

Arsenic is used commercially in many forms of insecticide, agricultural sprays, and especially by workers in grape vineyards. Its use as a medication is less popular now than formerly but still has advocates in prescribers of Fowler's solution and certain well-supported mail-order anti-asthmatic concoctions. Occupations which permit exposure to arsenic include paint or lacquer making, dye handling, leather handling and tanning, welding, cement making, canning, soap and candle manufacturing, lithography, and ink making.

PAGET'S DISEASE

About 3 per cent of people over 40 years of age have Paget's disease of bone (osteitis deformans). The pathologic features of bone destruction with formation of irregular new bone account for the variety of bizarre skeletal forms that result. As bone destruction and regeneration occur in close tandem there is no adherence to the original architectural design. As the bones become enlarged and distorted the increase in the circumference of the head may require a change in hat size, and the hands also tend to become larger and irregular in outline. The hands are frequently tender and exhibit a distinct tendency to fractures from even minor injuries.

TURNER'S SYNDROME

An interesting rather than important deviation of the morphologic structure of the hand occurs in Turner's syndrome (also called

Turner-Varney's syndrome, Albright's syndrome, ovarian agenesis, rudimentary ovary syndrome, and ovarian aplasia). It is a relatively uncommon syndrome and is characterized by several developmental defects of bodily structure. These include a short, thick-set stature, sexual infantilism, webbed neck, shield-shaped chest, widely spaced nipples, and cubitus valgus. The latter refers to the exaggerated angle at which the forearm is carried on the arm when the extremity is held at the sides.

The hand participates in the physical features of this curious syndrome by an abnormal lateral extension of the fifth finger which splays out from the others in a characteristic manner. Epiphyseal closure is delayed and syndactyly or polydactyly is frequently seen. Anomalous positioning of the fingers or toes is not uncommon.

High titers of urinary gonadotropins differentiate this syndrome from other forms of hypogonadism in which many of the physical characteristics of Turner's syndrome may be seen.

HURLER'S SYNDROME (Gargoylism)

Hurler's syndrome is a metabolic, genetically determined disturbance, perhaps related to the intracellular deposition of a mucopolysaccharide, which affects the skeleton and soft tissues. Among the outstanding features of this syndrome are clouding of the corneas, hepatosplenomegaly, mental deficiency, dwarfism, and skeletal changes.

The joints demonstrate a limitation of extensibility, especially prominent in the hands and fingers. The hands are wider than they are long and the fingers are held in a claw position. The fourth and fifth fingers are in-curved, much like the in-curving seen in mongolian idiocy.

7 *infections of the* HAND

Because of its wide range of operation in man's contact with work and play, and its unique position of vulnerability, the hand is exceptionally susceptible to trauma. This is substantiated by a statistical analysis which shows that the hand is the most frequently injured part of the body. Similarly, it is a common site for entry of numerous microorganisms, many of which are introduced through accidental inoculation by puncture wounds, lacerations, and other kinds of injury. Several specific infectious processes begin in this manner, and at times the pattern of invasion and the appearance of the resultant reaction is of value in its identification.

A consideration of infective disorders which have only local effects are not in context with this presentation. These include the various types of paronychia, felon, abscess, and cellulitis in the different anatomic compartments which call for a surgical orientation and are described in appropriate locations in the literature.

Certain other infections are limited to the hand as it represents a part of the total cutaneous organ, such as those related to several kinds of fungi or contact dermatitides which have little or no constitutional implication.

Most of the systemic mycotic diseases and the chronic granulomatous disorders may, and frequently do, produce inflammatory signs in the hand at the point of a break in the skin. Usually the configuration and behavior of many of these lesions resemble the classic chancre. Such is the case in sporotrichosis, actinomycosis, tuberculosis, syphilis, coccidiomycosis, tularemia, leishmaniasis, and blastomycosis, all of which are manifest by a papular or chancre-like lesion at the site of primary inoculation. Subsequently, the pathogenetic mechanism moves along more or less disease-specific and divergent pathways.

Fig. 115. Tuberculous chancre. Inoculation tuberculosis on the hand. Note secondary involvement of axillary lymph node. (Courtesy of Ormsby and Montgomery: Diseases of the Skin, 7th ed. Lea & Febiger.)

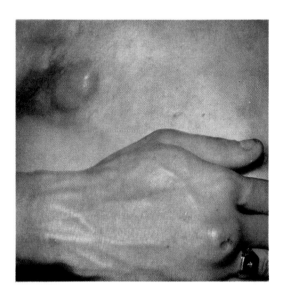

The need for careful and detailed history-taking is emphasized when an inflammatory lesion on the hand is encountered. Correlation with the environmental history is extremely helpful in assigning a proper diagnosis to this type of clinical finding. Information about accidental exposure to pathogens in occupation, sport, or hobby may offer considerable aid in discovering the cause for obscure systemic infections.

Some of the more prominent examples of constitutional infections which may exhibit associated signs in the hand, or frequently use the hand as a portal of entry, are included in this chapter.

TUBERCULOSIS

Two forms of cutaneous tuberculosis are of importance insofar as the hand is concerned. One is the primary tuberculous complex, the so-called tuberculous chancre, and the second is tuberculous verrucosa cutis.

A red nodule may form on a finger or on the dorsum of the hand, which is an equivalent to the Ghon lesion, and which represents a form of primary inoculation tuberculosis. It closely resembles the luetic extragenital chancre, or a furuncle. Like the Ghon complex, it represents the patient's first exposure to tuberculosis, and consequently is seen more often among children or in previously uninfected tuberculin-negative adults. As the initial nodular lesion ages it becomes indurated, may ulcerate, and is loaded with tubercle bacilli. After one or several months an associated lymphangitis appears, and the regional lymph nodes become enlarged. In this latter respect it may be differentiated from secondary inoculation forms of tuberculosis which are also noted not infrequently on the hand.

Secondary tuberculous lesions occur on the hands in persons who have active pulmonary tuberculosis (tuberculin positive) who inoculate the skin of their hands, usually the dorsum, by wiping their mouths. Acute inflammatory involvement of the lymphatic chain does not occur in secondary cutaneous tuberculous infection, but the regional nodes are enlarged.

Another type of infection occurs in persons who have been inoculated with the tubercle bacillus through an abrasion or wound on the hand. Tuberculous verrucosa cutis is found chiefly among workers in slaughterhouses or in the autopsy or dissection rooms and usually, therefore, in males. It appears as a papular or papulopustular lesion at the site of the inoculum, usually on the dorsum of the hand from whence it may extend to involve the forearm. It is extremely rare on the palms.

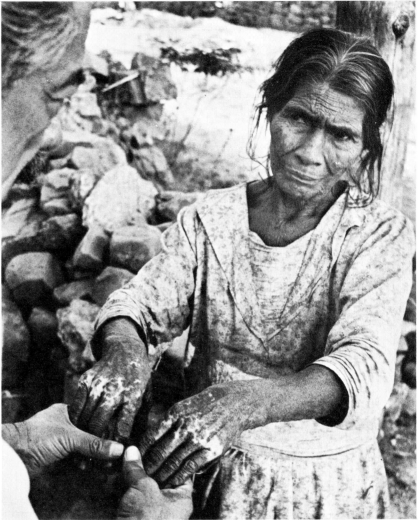

Fig. 116. Pinta. Depigmented areas in the skin of the hands in a patient with pinta (Mal de Pinto). (Courtesy of Bernard Cole: Roche Medical Image, April 1962.)

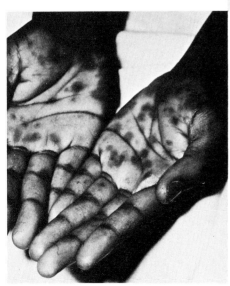

Fig. 117. Secondary syphilis. Macular rash on the palms in secondary syphilis. (Courtesy of John Lentz, M.D., Lankenau Hospital, Philadelphia.)

A more extensive involvement may be seen in which the lesions are warty, nodular and hyperkeratotic plaques with an irregular but clearly defined outline. A brick- or rust-colored crust may form on the surface. The lesions of tuberculous verrucosa cutis usually heal of their own accord and leave atrophic scars, hyperkeratoses, or irregular pigmentations.

Of some interest is the appearance of pitting in the nails of persons who are actively infected with tuberculosis. Hahn reports the finding in 100 per cent of his patients. Pitting was seen in only 6 per cent of patients whose disease had been inactive for a short time, and was absent in those who had shown no activity of tuberculous infection for more than one year.

Clubbing of the digits, the classic hippocratic fingers, has been associated with chronic pulmonary tuberculosis for centuries. It has been found in as many as 76 per cent of patients with pulmonary tuberculosis. Sometimes associated with the classic phthisic habitus are the thickened nails or longitudinal curving of the nail plate. Absence of the lunulae is sometimes encountered, and in certain patients cyanosis of the distal tips of the nails may occur.

SYPHILIS

The clinician must be alerted to the possibility that an ill-defined cutaneous lesion on the hand may represent a syphilitic infection. The most common site for the appearance of an extragenital chancre is on the finger. Similar to the type of primary sore seen on the skin or mucous membranes of the genitalia, digital chancres develop painlessly, approximately three weeks after inoculation. They become indurated with the passage of time, and ultimately assume the characteristics of an indolent, eroded lesion. Dark-field examination of smears from these lesions will establish the diagnosis. A discrete regional lymphadenitis, epitrochlear or axillary, is usually associated with the primary lesion.

The skin of the palm, being of a different structure than that of other parts of the body, does not favor the development of the usual maculopapular lesions of secondary syphilis. Instead, when a palmar syphiloderm occurs (the dorsums are only very rarely involved) the skin may be irregularly spotted with dull red macules which are covered with shaggy scales. Early in its course the rash is symmetric but later the lesion of each hand progresses independently with epidermal thickening, cracking, and peeling. The process may spread to the lateral surface of the hands, fingers, and wrists but has characteristically sharply defined edges where it meets the healthy skin.

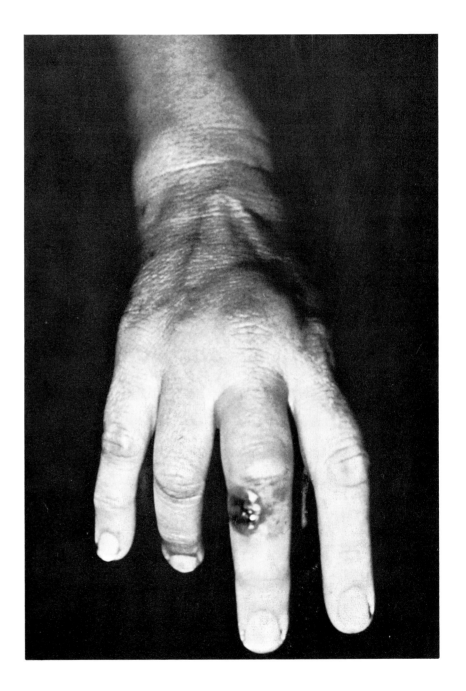

Fig. 118. Anthrax. Characteristic lesion on finger in "woolsorter's" disease.

SYPHILITIC DACTYLITIS

Syphilitic dactylitis is an infrequent manifestation of hereditary syphilis found in infants, usually between the third and seventh months of life. It represents an osteoperiostitis and is characterized clinically by a spindle-shaped involvement of the entire phalanx. It is usually not tender or painful. The lesion gradually increases in size but seldom suppurates, and the process is reversible by constitutional treatment.

ANTHRAX

The lesion of anthrax most often occurs on the exposed skin surfaces, particularly on the hands or neck and face. Malignant pustule, a term applied to the cutaneous hall-mark of anthrax, develops as a result of inoculation of spores in the skin, frequently through the agency of infected dust.

The characteristic lesion is a carbuncle or papule which has a black center and is surrounded by a halo of vesicles and inflammatory edema. Since the anthrax spores originate in animal sources, the history of exposure to potentially infected material is important. Thus, it is largely an occupational disease occurring in handlers of hides or carcasses of infected animals. Although anthrax usually is a cutaneous affliction, a less frequent means of entry is through inhalation of infected material which causes a pneumonic inflammation, usually rapidly fatal.

TULAREMIA

Tularemia is a bacterial infection caused by Pasteurella tularensis, which usually gains entry through the skin of the hand or finger, often through the slightest wound, by contact with an infected animal. Often the inoculum is introduced by the bite of a rodent, frequently a wild rabbit or a squirrel. Many other ground animals, such as the coyote and gopher and even the domestic cat, may carry the organism. Animals and blood-sucking insects, such as wood ticks or deer flies, which have bitten infected animals may be the means of spread of this infection. Tularemia is often seen among hunters or people who dress wild game.

The primary lesion is a papule which later becomes pustular. As the top of the nodule softens and sloughs, a dark necrotic plug is formed which eventually separates and leaves a punched-out, indolent ulcer. This cutaneous form of tularemia, the ulceroglandular type, usually begins in this fashion on the finger. Lymphangitis generally follows and causes enlargement of the regional lymph nodes which in turn may swell and form subcutaneous abscesses.

When an acute febrile illness is associated with an infected wound on the finger or hand, and a characteristic nodular lymphangitis and painful axillary adenopathy are combined with a history of possible exposure, the diagnosis of tularemia is suggested.

Tularemia must be differentiated from sporotrichosis.

SPOROTRICHOSIS

A widely distributed fungus, Sporotrichum schenckii, which is found on flowers, vegetables, plants, and shrubbery, particularly the barberry bush, is responsible for a systemic granulomatous infection, sporotrichosis. Characteristically, it produces a hard, spherical, movable nodule in the subcutaneous tissues of the hand, the so-called "sporotrichotic chancre." Florists, farmers, and gardeners, by virtue of their frequent exposure, are most often infected. Gumma-like nodules form an abscess which ultimately discharges a gelatinous type of pus and eventually develops into dark, granulomatous, necrotic ulcers. Inflammation and cording of the lymphatics draining the area extend up the arm to the axillary nodes. Of outstanding diagnostic importance is the characteristic string of discrete palpable nodules which form along the superficial lymphatic chain in the wrist and forearm. These painless, nodular lesions become attached to the overlying skin and may ulcerate. Indolent ulcerations and abscesses may spread and persist for years in the untreated patient. The organism is present in the ulcerated areas and can be cultured from the necrotic material, but is not usually visible in the lesions.

ACTINOMYCOSIS

The ray fungus enters a wound, often small and superficial, which may heal initially only to become the site of inflammatory activity after weeks or even months. A papule which resembles a small, cutaneous tumor forms in the skin, often in the hand. Eventually, at the site of the papule, an abscess develops which opens onto the skin surface through one or more sinus tracts. The purulent discharge contains "sulfur granules" which are identifiable microscopically as the thread-like fungus, Actinomyces. If untreated the infection progresses by undermining the skin and attacks the deeper tissues and bone.

BLASTOMYCOSIS

Cutaneous blastomycosis occurs on the hand or other exposed parts of the skin surface. It is due to invasion by a specific yeast fungus through a minor wound and is found most often in males who work outdoors and who are exposed to "earthy" jobs (farmers, cattle-handlers). The primary lesion is at first a non-tender papule which later becomes pustular. As it progresses, the superficial abscess breaks down and discharges mucopus in which the fungi are found. The lesion spreads in a roughly concentric fashion with the growing edge appearing as an angry, heaped-up, sloping rim. The base of the ulcer exhibits a tendency to heal centrally. Tiny deep-seated abscesses are studded around the advancing edge.

Systemic blastomycosis causes serious pulmonary and osseous invasive disease.

TETANUS

A lingering memory of a childhood playmate's unexpected death has contributed to a deep personal respect for the virulence of tetanus infection. My little friend was the neighborhood's marble-shooting champion, and was proud of the tough callus displayed on the middle knuckle, the accepted proof of his experience. In retrospect, it is all too obvious an invitation to tragedy—suitable environmental exposure and a portal sufficiently ajar.

Once inside, Clostridium tetani grows anaerobically. The wound itself is not remarkable in appearance but there is a vague subjective "drawing sensation" in and around it and later the muscles nearby become crampy. Muscular excitability and reflex irritability advance rapidly to trismus ("lockjaw"), opisthotonos, and striking manifestations of other skeletal muscle spasms and contractions.

Puncture wounds, however small, sustained in the vicinity of the stable, the garden, or the athletic field, or those incurred by tines or nails, rusty or not, must be viewed with great urgency, particularly among the non-immunized.

TRICHINIASIS

The classic physical finding in the hand of the patient with trichiniasis is the appearance of splinter hemorrhages under the nails. They are roughly triangular-shaped petechiae which are arranged in transverse rows at the same distance from the free edge in all the nails.

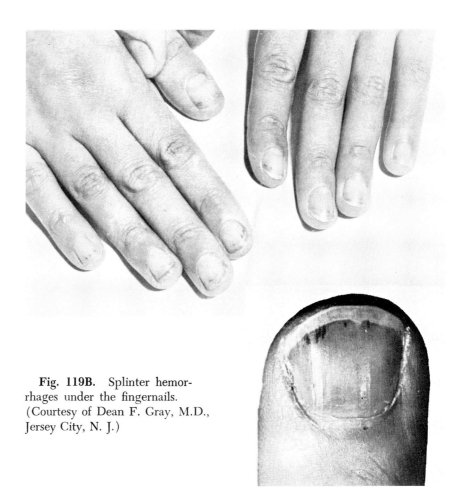

Fig. 119A. Trichiniasis. Splinter hemorrhages are found under the fingernails in 60 to 70 per cent of individuals infested with Trichina. The presence of eosinophilia, conjunctival edema and splinter hemorrhages in the same patient is sufficient to establish a diagnosis of trichiniasis. (Courtesy of J. G. Downing, M.D.: Cutaneous Manifestations of Systemic Disease. Charles C Thomas.)

Fig. 119B. Splinter hemorrhages under the fingernails. (Courtesy of Dean F. Gray, M.D., Jersey City, N. J.)

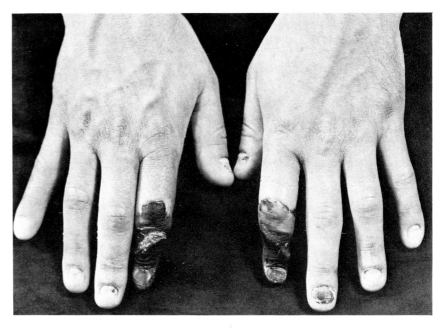

Fig. 120. Raynaud's phenomenon. Gangrene of the index fingers in Raynaud's phenomenon. (Courtesy of G. de Takats, M.D., and E. F. Fowler, M.D.: J.A.M.A. 179:103.)

The flat edges of the hemorrhagic fringe face distally and the apex points toward the lunula. It is thought that splinter hemorrhages are due to larval emboli.

Numbness of the digits is common in cases of porkworm infestation. Excessive perspiration, periorbital edema, suffusion of the conjunctivae, eosinophilia, and subungual petechiae are signs which suggest strongly the diagnosis of trichiniasis.

Similar splinter hemorrhages are seen in subacute bacterial endocarditis, rheumatic fever, and in blood dyscrasias of certain types which are accompanied by bleeding tendencies. Subungual hemorrhages, more irregular in outline, are seen in Rendu-Osler-Weber's disease (hemorrhagic familial telangiectasia) and in scurvy.

Infestation with hookworm has been accompanied by burning sensations in the palms, and ascariasis may cause an eczematous rash on the hands.

GANGRENE OF THE FINGERTIPS

Dry gangrene of one or all the fingertips may complicate numerous severe systemic infections such as meningitis, malaria, typhus fever, typhoid fever, scarlet fever, diphtheria, pneumonia, and severe bacteremias. Instances of irreversible vasospasm due to prolonged intravenous infusion of levoarterenol or other vasopressor agents, used therapeutically in the management of circulatory failure, have been responsible for the development of gangrene in the fingers.

Severe Raynaud's phenomenon, with development of gangrene of the fingertips, has been associated with periarteritis nodosa. The occurrence of digital gangrene may proceed from vascular interference at any level along the course of the arterial supply such as occurs in aneurysm, scalenus anticus syndrome, cervical rib, or in sclerotic, spastic, embolic, or thrombotic occlusive disease.

LEPROSY

The long, smoldering course of leprosy, which continues for many years before death occurs, permits the development of severe deformities, some of which are incredibly grotesque. Pathologic effects are widespread in the body, but only those which involve the hand will be considered here.

One of the earliest signs is anhidrosis of the fingertips and, with progression of the disease, anesthesia of one or more fingers begins. Although initially the anesthesia may be limited to a single digit,

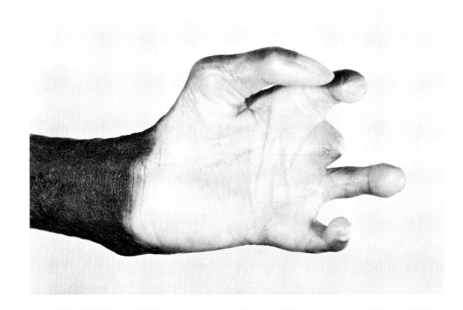

Fig. 121. Leper's hand. Resorption of phalanges and paralysis in a patient with moderately advanced leprosy. (Courtesy of Edgar B. Johnwick, Carville, La.)

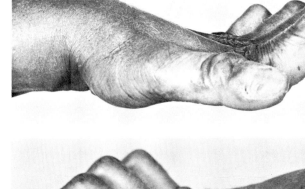

Fig. 122 A & B. Leprosy. Peripheral nerve involvement in a leper is a common early sign. Characteristic anesthesia and motor weakness of the ulnar and median nerves are present in this patient. Note atrophic effects in the musculature and claw-hand deformity. (Courtesy of Edgar B. Johnwick, Carville, La.)

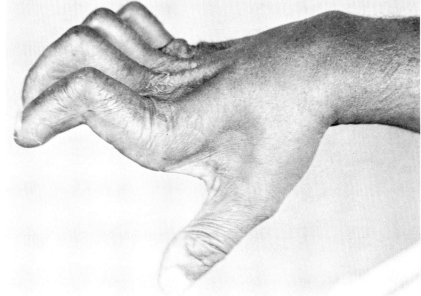

eventually the characteristic acroanesthesia becomes symmetric in its distribution. Such symmetric involvement is an outstanding feature of leprosy. Absence of perception of thermal or other painful trauma leads ultimately to ulcerations of the fingers and changes in skin pigmentation. White-skinned persons show gray or brown pigmentations on the hands and elsewhere where leprous invasion has occurred, whereas depigmentation is observed in the dark-skinned races.

Muscular atrophies are common, and are related to neural damage in the leper. As a result of atrophy, which demonstrates a special affinity for the small muscles of the hand, claw-like contracture deformities occur.

Fingernails become atrophic, deformed, and often disappear. Resorption of bones, especially of the phalanges, leads to mutilation and seriously disabling auto-amputations of the digits. The middle phalanx may disappear first and secondary infections are frequent. Progressive circulatory and inflammatory disease eventuates in acral gangrene, adding to the over-all destruction of the hands.

RUBELLA

A self-limited type of polyarthritis may occur as a complication of rubella or German measles. The small and medium-sized joints of the hand, wrists, and ankles have been affected with swelling and arthralgia which lasts for about a week.

8

diseases of the NAILS

Deranged morphology of the fingernails is observed in many severe systemic disorders largely through the mechanism of interference with the normal nutritional and growth properties of the nail. Alterations in the appearance and structure of the nail attend a variety of generalized disorders such as anemic states, dietary deficiencies, dysendocrinisms, drug or chemical toxicity, circulatory disorders, infectious diseases, and certain degenerative conditions. As a result of these diversified etiologic factors the nails may demonstrate structural alterations which include splitting, shedding or separation of the nail plate, ridging, thinning, striation, or any type of surface irregularity. In certain instances the abnormalities of the nails may occur early in the course of a systemic disease, occasionally as a sentinel sign of an insidiously advancing general disease. Evidences of unusual wear in characteristic parts of the nail or the presence of stains provide broad clues to occupational associations.

Although subject to wide differences in health, the average daily adult nail growth is approximately 0.1 millimeters. In pregnancy, in warmer climates, and in nail-biters there is an increased rate of nail growth. Measles, the common cold, septicemia, and other acute infections are capable of interrupting the normal growth of nails. Patients afflicted with malnutrition, nephrosis, and many systemic chronic diseases frequently have a retarded rate of growth of nails, although there is not universal acceptance of this concept. When arrest or retardation of growth in the nail occurs, either as the result of local or systemic nutritional effects, transverse bands or ridges appear in the surface of the plate.

In peripheral vascular disease there is a retardation of nail and hair growth in the deficient extremity or part of an extremity, while

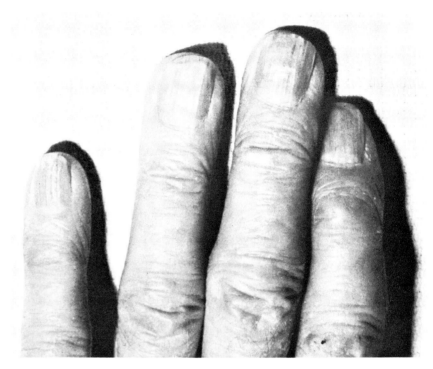

Fig. 123. Ridged nails. Thickened, vertically ridged and irregular nails in one hand, due to trophic changes secondary to cervical osteoporosis and nerve root damage.

Fig. 124. Nail-biting (onychophagia). Severely bitten nails in an adult male. Such neurotic practices have no known harmful effects and are quite common among children until about the age of puberty. The presence of the habit among adults usually indicates a somewhat higher order of neurosis and is apparently related to tension states. The patient pictured above had had two major surgical procedures for bleeding peptic ulcer by age 22 years.

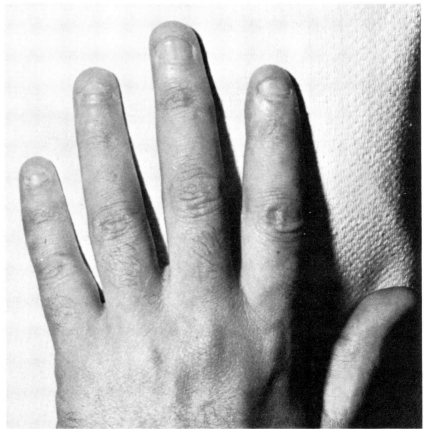

an increased blood flow or chronic hyperemia enhances hair and nail development. Chronic hyperemia is observed in mentally defective individuals who are "hand suckers." A localized oval hyperemic area is produced by habitual sucking, frequently at a site on the dorsum of the hand. In the same location, hyperpigmentation and a long luxuriant hair growth develops due to the effects of hyperemia.

Emotional disturbances, acute or long endured, may leave their marks in the nails in the form of superficial pitting of the nail plate, thinning or splitting and, in some instances, causes separation of the nail from its bed (neuronychia). Nail-biting and cuticle-picking are well-known neurotic habits.

COLOR CHANGES IN THE NAILS

Cyanosis in the tissues, particularly prominent in the nail beds and on the tips of the extremities, is related to an increased amount of reduced hemoglobin or derivatives of hemoglobin. Whenever blood flow to the hands is reduced, either as a systemic or local defect, cyanosis generally occurs. It may also appear if the venous return is impeded. If cyanosis is present in a warm hand a systemic cause rather than a local one is suspected, such as occurs in acute or chronic pulmonary disorders or in errors of pulmonic diffusion. Certain other mechanisms may less frequently account for color changes in the fingers and such changes must be distinguished from the blueness due to circulatory deficits.

Cyanotic fingers will blanch when blood is expressed from the tissues by pressure, whereas other pigments will remain. The severely anemic individual may be incapable of demonstrating cyanosis because of an absolute diminished amount of hemoglobin available. Conversely, the polycythemic individual may display cyanosis even in the absence of any other demonstrable circulatory abnormality, because of increased concentrations of hemoglobin.

Quinacrine, camoquin, phenolphthalein, sodium nitrate, and nitrites are capable of causing a deep-blue discoloration in the fingertips and a plum color in the capillary blood. Silver deposits in the extremities (argyria) are fixed in the tissues and will not blanch out with pressure. Enterogenous cyanosis results when methemoglobin and sulfhemoglobin accumulate in the body as occurs after exposure to hydrogen sulfide. Some of the older sulfonamide compounds, little-used in therapy today, such as sulfanilamide and sulfapyridine, can produce a blueness of the mucous membranes, nail beds, and fingertips.

Not so commonly now as in the past, several of the patent medicines, particularly headache powders, contained a most effective

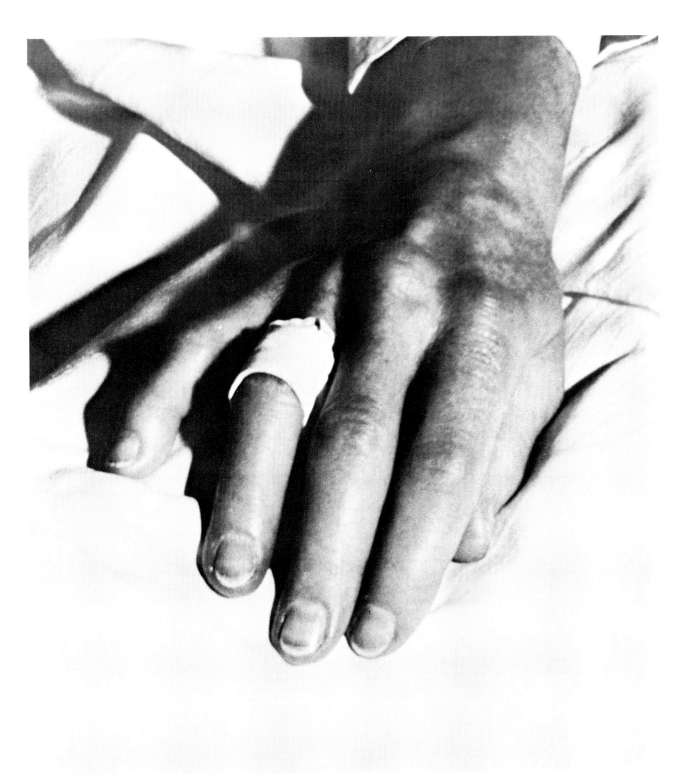

Fig. 125. Polycythemia. Cyanosis of the hand and nails in a patient with polycythemia. Color blanches partially with pressure. Note intensification of duskiness at the distal rim of the nail bed.

analgesic, acetanilid, which caused a blueness in the skin. Fortunately, the grape-juice appearance of the blood and the cyanosis in the skin are promptly correctable upon withdrawal of the drug.

In cyanotic heart disease, when mixing of blood from the right and left sides of the heart occurs, there are physical changes in the hand that are dramatically reversible when surgical correction is effected. Clubbed fingers, cyanosis, and polycythemia in a very young child suggest a cardiac etiologic factor. Clubbing without cyanosis, when observed in a child, should prompt a search for an extracardiac cause.

The azure lunulae of Wilson's disease (hepatolenticular degeneration) are due to the deposition of copper in the moons of the nails. This condition and the dark yellow nails of the patient with Addison's disease and the white nails seen in the patient with cirrhosis have been mentioned elsewhere in this text.

MEE'S LINES

Grooves or ridges and transverse lines of a light or dark color are seen frequently in the fingernails under a variety of stressful situations. Whether we identify them as Beau's lines or Mee's lines, or white bands, their occurrence appears to be related in all instances to a localized nutritional derangement.

The germinal portion of the nail is supersensitive to stress, such as infection, fever, toxicities (arsenic and thallium), deficiency states, traumas (either local or constitutional), and perhaps even emotional upsets. Following surgical procedures or severe illnesses, the nutrition of the nail (and other cutaneous structures) is disturbed. Often such disturbance is visible as a change in the nail being formed at the time of the insult, so that it grows out as a light or dark transverse band, or an indentation of the nail plate. As the nail continues to grow, the band or groove travels along with it. It is often possible to estimate the date of an infection or surgical procedure by measuring the distance of these marks from the lunula. The average rate of nail growth in the healthy adult is approximately one millimeter in every 10 days.

The occurrence of bands and grooves in the nails under these circumstances has been described in medical literature for many generations. Vogel, in 1870, drew sketches of grooved nails in a patient with typhus fever. They are sometimes observed in patients with Hodgkin's granuloma.

Paired white bands on the third and fourth fingernails bilaterally, which are neither palpable nor indented, have been described in association with hypoalbuminemia.

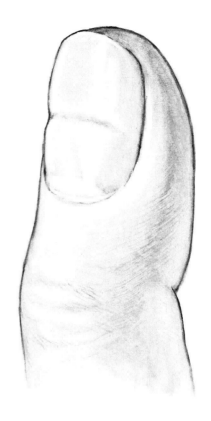

Fig. 126. Beau's line. Transverse groove which is related to a nutritional disturbance in the nail plate. Severe systemic infections or poisoning (thallium, drugs, etc.) may be causal factors.

Fig. 127. Mee's lines. Transverse white lines which appeared in the nails of an individual at the time of a massive myocardial infarction. (Three months after his attack, when this photograph was taken, the lines had grown out to the middle of the nail.)

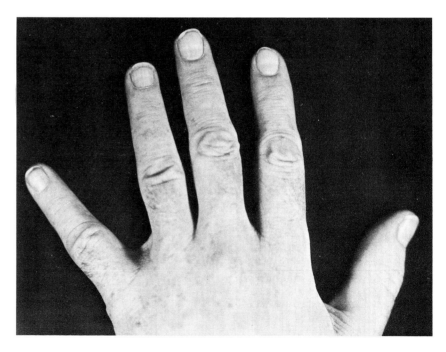

BEAU'S LINES

Transverse ridges appear in the nail under circumstances of impaired nutrition, due either to local or systemic conditions. These ridges or lines (Beau's lines) begin at the lunula and move toward the periphery as the nail grows outward. Nervous shocks, chronic alcoholism, accidental trauma, infections, high fevers, surgical procedures, and many other diverse stressful situations may cause the development of these changes in the nails. Since it takes approximately six months for a nail to grow out completely, and a shorter time being required in warm environments, the date of onset of the nutritional defect may be roughly estimated by observation of the location of the furrow and noting its distance from the lunula.

HYPOALBUMINEMIA

The presence of paired narrow white bands in the fingernails has been found in association with low levels of serum albumin. This phenomenon occurs in patients afflicted with a variety of disease states in which the serum albumin is found to be persistently below 2.2 grams per 100 ml.

The white bands are arranged parallel with the lunula and are neither palpable nor indented. They are separated from one another and from the lunula by thin strips of normal-appearing pink nail. Sometimes the distal band is slightly wider than the other one. Originally described in the nails of nephrotic individuals, these bands may be present in patients with any condition in which hypoalbuminemia is associated.

GLOSSARY OF NAIL PATHOLOGY

Condition	Description	Occurrence
Beau's lines	Transverse lines or ridges marking repeated disturbances of nail growth	Systemic diseases, toxic or nutritional deficiency states of many types; trauma (from manicuring)
Defluvium unguium (Onychomadesis)	Complete loss of nails	Certain systemic diseases such as scarlet fever, syphilis, leprosy, alopecia areata, and exfoliative dermatitis
Diffusion of lunula unguis	"Spreading" of lunula	Dystrophies of the extremities

Condition	Description	Occurrence
Eggshell nails	Nail plate thin, semi-transparent, bluish-white, with a tendency to curve upward at the distal edge	Syphilis
Fragilitas unguium	Friable or brittle nails	Dietary deficiency, local trauma, conditions caused by contact with chemical agents; syphilis and other systemic diseases
Hapalonychia	Nails very soft, split easily	Following contact with strong alkalis; endocrine disturbances, malnutrition, syphilis, chronic arthritis
Hippocratic nails	"Watch-glass nails" associated with "drumstick fingers"	Chronic respiratory and circulatory diseases, especially pulmonary tuberculosis; hepatic cirrhosis
Koilonychia	"Spoon nails," nails are concave on the outer surface	In dysendocrinisms (acromegaly), trauma, dermatoses, syphilis, nutritional deficiencies, hypochromic anemias, hypothyroidism
Leukonychia	White spots or striations or rarely the whole nail may turn white (congenital type)	Local trauma, hepatic cirrhosis, nutritional deficiencies and many systemic diseases
Mee's lines	Transverse white bands	Hodgkin's granuloma, arsenical and thallium toxicity, high fevers, local nutritional derangement
Moniliasis of nails	Infection (usually paronychia) caused by yeast forms (Candida albicans)	Frequently in food-handlers, dentists, dishwashers, gardeners
Onychatrophia	Atrophy or failure of development of nails	Trauma, infection, dysendocrinism, gonadal aplasia, and many systemic diseases
Onychauxis	Nail plate is greatly thickened	Mild persistent trauma, systemic diseases such as peripheral stasis, peripheral neuritis, syphilis, leprosy, hemiplegia, or at times may be congenital
Onychia	Inflammation of the nail matrix causing deformity of the nail plate	Trauma, infection, many systemic diseases
Onychodystrophy	Any deformity of the nail plate, nail bed, or nail matrix	Many diseases; trauma; or may be caused by chemical agents (poisoning, allergy)
Onychogryposis	"Claw nails"—extreme degree of hypertrophy, sometimes with horny projections arising from the nail surface	May be congenital or related to many chronic systemic diseases (see onychauxis above)
Onycholysis	Loosening of the nail plate beginning at the distal or free edge	Trauma, injury by chemical agents, many systemic diseases, hyperthyroidism

Condition	Description	Occurrence
Onychomadesis	Shedding of all the nails (defluvium unguium)	Dermatoses such as exfoliative dermatitis, alopecia areata, psoriasis, eczema, nail infection, severe systemic diseases, arsenical poisoning
Onychophagia	Nail biting	Neurosis
Onychorrhexis	Longitudinal ridging and splitting of the nails	Dermatoses, nail infections, many systemic diseases, senility, injury by chemical agents, and hyperthyroidism
Onychoschizia	Lamination and scaling away of nails in thin layers	Dermatoses, syphilis, injury by chemical agents
Onychotillomania	Alteration of the nail structures caused by persistent neurotic picking at the nails	Neurosis
Pachyonychia	Extreme thickening of all the nails. The nails are more solid and more regular than in onychogryposis	Usually congenital and associated with hyperkeratosis of the palms and soles
Pterygium unguis	Thinning of the nail fold and spreading of the cuticle over the nail plate	Associated with vasospastic conditions such as Raynaud's phenomenon and occasionally with hypothyroidism

(Slightly modified after C. J. White)

9

Dermatoglyphics

It is highly unlikely that any patient has ever thought to inquire as to the reason behind a physician's inspection of his oral cavity, conjunctivae, or chest. However, the usual reaction of a patient who becomes aware that his hands are the object of close scrutiny by an examining physician follows a predictable sequence of inquisitiveness. Perhaps this is due to the traditional mental associations that link the study of palms with fortune telling or charlatanism in carnival tents. This attitude persists in spite of an increasing interest in medical investigation that has placed dermatoglyphics in an important position as a valuable aid in psychologic evaluation and, more recently, as a point in the differentiation of congenital and acquired cardiac malformation. The numerous examples touched upon in this presentation show, I believe, how the presence of systemic disease can affect the appearance or function of the hand in one way or another.

From England, Charlotte Wolf carried her intensely scholarly interest in hand study to the asylums of the European continent where she pursued the question of hand configurations, development, expressiveness, and dermatoglyphic content as related to mentality, intellectual development, and psychologic behavior. Her work, published in 1951, lays an excellent understructure for scientific correlation of psychopathic disorders and endocrinopathic diseases with hand size, shape and function, and with the distribution, number and types of creases in the palms. By comparing the palmprints of many hundreds of mentally defective patients in several institutions with the "normal" pattern, a high level of correlation is evident, thus giving scientific approbation to earliest Aristotelian premises of hand and intellect relationships.

Not only is the type of lines and creases in the palms significant but also of interpretive value is a study of the length of the fingers as compared with the size of the palm and the size of digits relative to one another. The manner in which the thumb is joined to the palm and the structure of the nails and the complexities of gestures may all contribute to a clinical interpretation. For example, among the lower primates there is but a single crease traversing the palm. Creases form as a reflection of manual mobility involving certain parts of the hand and since the monkey cannot use his thumb or index finger individually the second transverse palmar crease is not present (Simian hand). Secondary or small accessory creases form in the palm according to the plasticity and the manner of use of the owner's hands so that considerably more importance is ascribed to the appearance, number and location of the smaller lines than to the major folds. The mentally defective individual who lacks dextrous hand function shows clearly such inadequacies in the hand which is poorly formed, and an incomplete and abnormal formation of the small accessory folds in the skin of the palm.

The mongolian idiot has a rudimentary fifth finger which is usually shorter than normal, curved inward toward the ring finger, and is used ineffectively and awkwardly. Consequently, this type of individual frequently lacks a second interphalangeal fold on the little finger. "The peculiar conformation of the hand in mongoloid idiots is certainly a developmental associate of variants in the dermatoglyphics. Perhaps some of the distinctions in the palmar dermatoglyphics are correlated specifically with the presence of a simian line, a modified transverse flexion crease coursing continuously from radial to ulnar margins of the palm. The simian line, occasional in normal persons, occurs quite frequently in mongolian idiots."

A short fifth finger has been associated in some instances with a behavior problem, although it has been noted as a familial trait in seemingly normal people.

Since the index finger and thumb complex make up the major structural deviation of the human hand from the lower animals closest to man, the morphology of these particular digits represents man's departure upward in the evolutionary scale. The middle finger is almost always the longest of the fingers, and either the index or the ring finger is the next longest. In the highly developed intellect the index finger, which represents the human digital formula, is frequently long and well developed.

The length of the fifth finger is increased out of normal proportions quite often in schizophrenics. In the interpretation of hand shapes in mental disorders, the manner in which the thumb is set into the hand carries the highest percentage of correlation. The

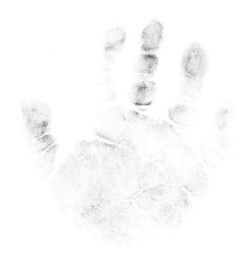

Fig. 128. Mongolism. Palm print showing incurved, shortened fifth finger and a *single* transverse palmar crease. Frequently only one transverse crease is found in the little finger, although this infant has two.

Fig. 129A. Familial sclero-dactyly. Hand-type is genetically conditioned. This 86-year-old male has a stiff, only partially mobile hand which, because of limited flexibility since birth, demonstrates a simple crease-pattern in the palms and fingers. Note single transverse palmar crease and poorly delineated digital folds.

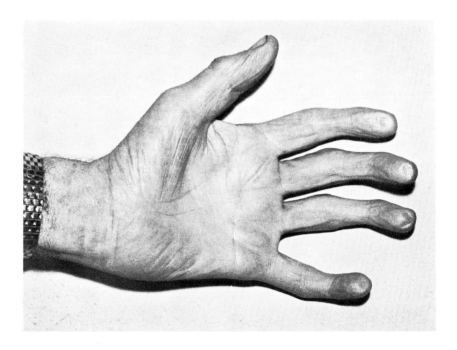

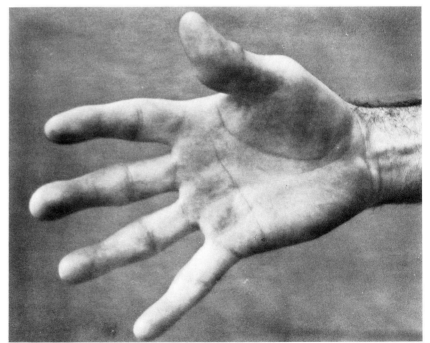

Fig. 129B. The son of the above individual has the same hand-type, including a single palmar transverse crease and a single digital crease.

so-called "simian insertion" of the thumb, in which the digit is located well back toward the wrist, and at a more or less right angle with the hand, invariably connotes a pathologic mentality. The reliability of this sign is reputed to be 100 per cent. The absence of the second crease in the fifth finger has similar significance in the association with mental disease. Concave nails or immature development of the nails and cuticular structures also portend an inferior intellect and rank high among the congenital deformities to be noted in the hands of the mentally defective. An abnormally short fifth finger or thumb which may occasionally be found among normal people is, however, a physical aberration which carries a high index of suspicion in the probability of mental or behavioral deviations.

I have observed several examples of clubbed thumbs, a physical trait which bears the sanguine and imaginative term "murderer's thumb" in the language of chiromancy (see Fig. 78). Somewhat disappointingly, these individuals who were so stigmatized were exceptionally stable emotionally, and had chosen as their respective occupations such law-abiding fields as professional golf, high fashion modeling, medical secretaryship, and the like. Very often clubbed thumbs and other developmental variations in the finger and hand shape and size, as well as syndactylism, follow a strong heritable pattern, even in the absence of other major abnormal structural defects.

The comparison of palm prints must be made against a standard and there quite understandably can be no fixed "normal" because each hand has its own unique configuration of papillary ridges. Consequently, the comparison must be made between groups on the basis of frequency of certain patterns common to most "normals," using criteria established along the most general of variable standards. In the clinical employment of this index as in the internal systemic diseases, physical findings in the hand must be considered as mere adjuncts for the most part, and are useful principally as corroborative evidence in diagnosis. Dermatoglyphics, strictly defined, is a term applied to the finely sculptured patterns of the skin which appear on the palmar and plantar surfaces of the hand and foot. It is used, also, to designate the field of anatomic science concerned with the study of these configurations.

The highly specialized skin of the palm and sole is different from that which covers the rest of the body. The delicate corrugations which enhance friction and the gripping function are peculiar to these parts and serve the same general purpose as the tread on a tire. Another noteworthy difference in the skin of the palm is the absence of hair and sebaceous glands. Early in the second trimester

Fig. 130. Examples of triradii.

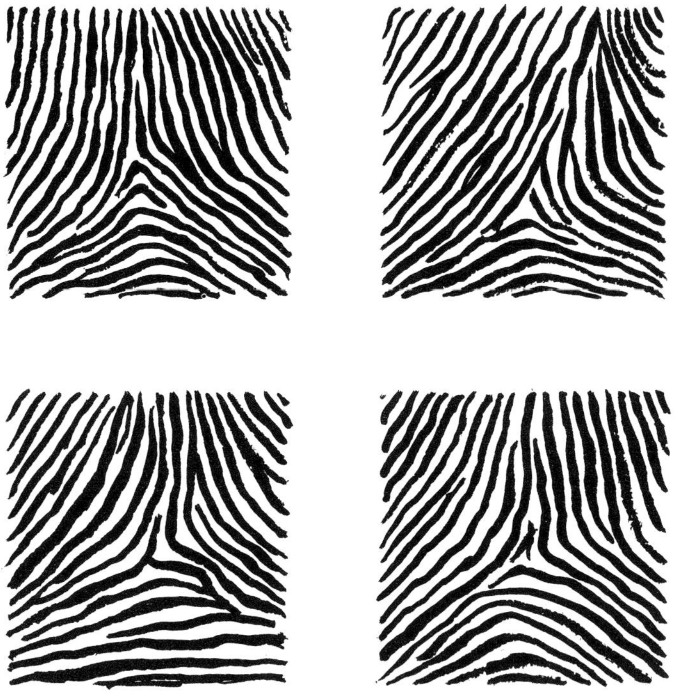

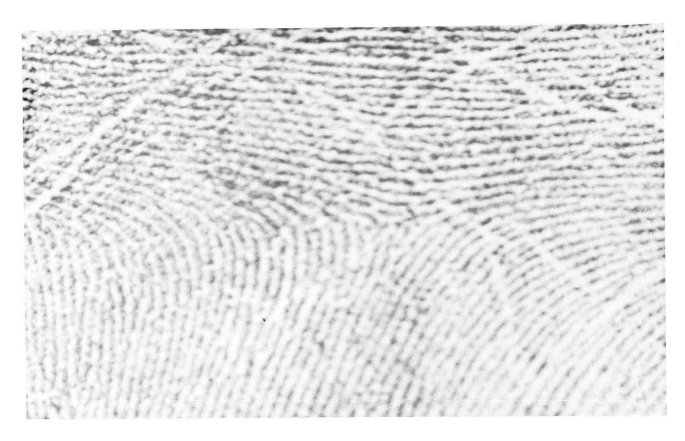

Fig. 131. Palm print showing triradius. Normal palm print showing delta-like configuration (triradius).

of pregnancy the process of formation of the complicated patterns, whorls, and ridges of the palmar skin of the fetus is initiated. The ultimate distinctive configuration of ridge systems evolves from germinal hubs in the thenar, hypothenar, interdigital and apical pads. As the gnurling pattern develops in the fetal hand and advances in crude centrifugal paths from the several centers, small delta-shaped configurations are formed where they come together. These formations are called triradii. Other anatomic defects in fetal development which occur at or about the same time may affect the formation of the ridge systems and thereby stigmatize the palm.

A triradius is a Y-shaped hub in the geometric pattern of ridges and grooves in the friction skin of the hand. It is located at the meeting point of three opposing ridge systems and has significance to the student of dermatoglyphics as a landmark for counting and mapping. The triradii are of various trispoked forms and occur in different areas in the hand, such as in the interdigital intervals in the palm (digital triradii) and the proximal margin of the palm (axial triradii). The axial triradii are situated in the general location of the axial fold between the hypothenar and thenar muscle masses and most commonly are in line with the fourth metacarpal bone. Recent studies have been directed toward correlating the location of axial triradii and the incidence of certain congenital deformities.

Usually there is only a single axial triradius quite close to the transverse ("bracelet") crease at the proximal limit of the palm. Occasionally, these triradii are multiple, two or even three, lying at different levels in the longitudinal axis. More rarely, there is no axial triradius present. The distal spoke of the axial triradius extends to become the main (axial) line, terminating, in most instances, between the thumb and index finger.

For a more extensive and scientific account of this subject the interested reader is referred to the monograph, "Fingerprints, Palms and Soles" by Cummins and Midlo (Blakiston Co., 1943).

When a topic such as "palm reading" ventures into the field of clinical medicine the first impulses stirred in the mind give less than full sanction. To be sure it is a delicate ground to tread upon in stepping into a discussion of what has been labeled the pseudo-science of dactyloscopy. The limitations are understandably many, but more interest and study are called for to better delineate the boundaries of what is or is not valid.

We may be on the threshold of new applications of clinical importance in the not-so-new science of dermatoglyphics. At Tulane University there appears to be an active center where an impetus has arisen suggesting that we take another look at its diagnostic potential in medicine.

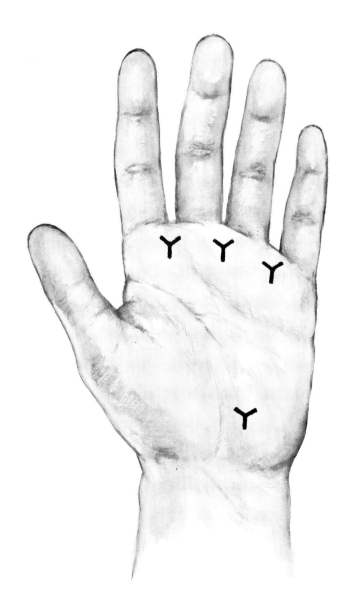

Fig. 132. Showing position of normal triradii. (A), Digital triradii. (B), Axial triradius.

A

B

Cummins records the palmar patterns and shows statistically significant deviations from "normal" among individuals with epilepsy, feeble-mindedness, idiocy (most noteworthy differences occur in mongolian idiots), and neurofibromatosis. Characteristic sex and racial differences, variations due to skin pigmentation, differences in body measurements, and other anthropologic and genetic variations are implied. An analysis of palm prints has been offered in court in litigation involving a paternity dispute. Judgment was passed, however, that such evidence was from an area of science yet insufficiently acceptable as proof of paternity. Dermatoglyphics are accepted as valid diagnostic criteria in distinguishing monozygotic and dizygotic twins.

Hale, Phillips and Burch ventured into scientific palm reading with conclusions which, although admittedly tentative, stamped their nihil obstat on the method. These investigators pointed out a relationship between the positioning of axial triradii in the palm, and a likelihood of a congenital malformation in the cardiac structures. In their patients with congenital cardiac defects the frequency of occurrence of a triradius distal to the t prime position, or the presence of multiple triradii was approximately double that found in a control group. Multiple axial triradii and distal displacement of the axial triradius occurred more often in patients whose cardiac lesion was congenital rather than acquired.

Most certainly this observation will stimulate further study of an interesting phenomenon so that still another tool is added to the evergrowing list of diagnostic methods which, refreshingly, does not require the use of highly specialized technical personnel or biotronic devices.

Outline of
PHYSICAL FINDINGS
IN THE HAND

VARIATIONS IN SIZE AND SHAPE OF HAND

large, blunt fingers (spade hand)
 acromegaly
 Hurler's disease (gargoylism)

gross irregularity of shape and size
 Paget's disease of bone
 Maffucci's syndrome
 neurofibromatosis

spider fingers, slender palm (arachnodactyly)
 Marfan's syndrome
 sickle cell disease
 pulmonic valve stenosis

slender, delicate, hyperextensible fingers
 hypopituitary
 eunuchism
 Ehlers-Danlos syndrome, pseudoxanthoma elasticum
 tuberculosis
 asthenic habitus
 osteogenesis imperfecta

sausage-shaped phalanges
 rickets (beading of joints)
 granulomatous dactylitis (tuberculosis, syphilis)

spindliform joints (fingers)
 early rheumatoid arthritis
 systemic lupus erythematosus

spindliform joints (fingers) (*continued*)
    psoriasis
    rubella
    Boeck's sarcoidosis
    osteoarthritis

cone-shaped fingers
    pituitary obesity
    Fröhlich's dystrophy adiposogenitalis

unilateral enlargement of hand
    arteriovenous aneurysm
    Maffucci's syndrome

square dry hands
    cretinism
    myxedema

single, widened, flattened distal phalanx
    sarcoidosis

shortened fourth and fifth metacarpals (brachymetacarpalia)
    pseudohypoparathyroidism
    pseudopseudohypoparathyroidism

shortened, incurved fifth finger (symptom of DuBois)
    mongolism
    "behavioral problem"
    gargoylism (broad, short, thick-skinned hand)

malposition and abduction, fifth finger
    Turner's syndrome (gonadal dysgenesis, webbed neck, etc.)

syndactylism
    congenital malformations of the heart, great vessels
    multiple congenital deformities
    Laurence-Moon-Biedl syndrome
    in normal individuals as an inherited trait

clubbed fingers
    subacute bacterial endocarditis
    pulmonary causes
        tuberculosis
        pulmonary arteriovenous fistula
        pulmonic abscess
        pulmonic cysts
        bullous emphysema
        pulmonary hypertrophic osteoarthropathy
        bronchogenic carcinoma

clubbed fingers (*continued*)
  alveolocapillary block
    interstitial pulmonary fibrosis
    sarcoidosis
    beryllium poisoning
    sclerodermatous lung
    asbestosis
    miliary tuberculosis
    alveolar cell carcinoma
  cardiovascular causes
    patent ductus arteriosus
    tetralogy of Fallot
    Taussig-Bing complex
    pulmonic stenosis
    ventricular septal defect
  diarrheal states
    ulcerative colitis
    tuberculous enteritis
    sprue
    amebic dysentery
    bacillary dysentery
    parasitic infestation (G-I tract)
  hepatic cirrhosis
  myxedema
  polycythemia
  chronic urinary tract infections (upper and lower)
    chronic nephritis
  hyperparathyroidism (telescopy of distal phalanx)
  pachydermoperiostosis (syndrome of Touraine, Solente and Golé)

joint disturbances
  arthritides
    osteoarthritis
    rheumatoid arthritis
    systemic lupus erythematosus
    gout
    psoriasis
    sarcoidosis
    endocrinopathy (acromegaly)
    rheumatic fever
    Reiter's syndrome
    dermatomyositis
  anaphylactic reaction—serum sickness
  scleroderma

EDEMA OF THE HAND

cardiac disease (congestive heart failure)

hepatic disease

renal disease
    nephritis
    nephrosis

hemiplegic hand

syringomyelia

superior vena caval syndrome
    superior thoracic outlet tumor
    mediastinal tumor or inflammation
    pulmonary apex tumor
    aneurysm

generalized anasarca, hypoproteinemia

postoperative lymphedema (radical breast amputation)

ischemic paralysis (cold, blue, swollen, numb)

lymphatic obstruction
    lymphomatous masses in axilla

axillary mass
    metastatic tumor, abscess, leukemia, Hodgkin's disease

aneurysm of ascending or transverse aorta, or of axillary artery

pressure on innominate or subclavian vessels

Raynaud's disease

myositis

cervical rib

trichiniasis

scalenus anticus syndrome

NEUROMUSCULAR EFFECTS

atrophy
    painless:
        amyotrophic lateral sclerosis
        Charcot-Marie-Tooth peroneal atrophy
        syringomyelia (loss of heat, cold and pain sensation)
        neural leprosy
    painful:
        peripheral nerve disease

atrophy (*continued*)
    painful (*continued*):
        peripheral nerve disease (*continued*)
            radial nerve (wrist drop)
                lead poisoning, alcoholism, polyneuritis, trauma, diphtheria, polyarteritis, neurosyphilis, anterior poliomyelitis
            ulnar nerve (benediction palsy)
                polyneuritis, trauma
            median nerve (claw hand)
                carpal-tunnel syndrome
                    rheumatoid arthritis
                    tenosynovitis at wrist
                    amyloidosis
                    gout
                    plasmacytoma
                    anaphylactic reaction
                    menopause syndrome
                    myxedema

extrinsic pressure on the nerve (cervical, axillary, supraclavicular or brachial)
    Pancoast tumor (pulmonary apex)
    aneurysms of subclavian arteries, axillary vessels, or thoracic aorta
    costoclavicular syndrome
    superior thoracic outlet syndrome
    cervical rib
    degenerative arthritis of cervical spine
    herniation of cervical intervertebral disk

shoulder-hand syndrome
    myocardial infarction
    Pancoast tumor
    brain tumor
    intrathoracic neoplasms
    discogenetic disease
    cervical spondylosis
    febrile panniculitis
    senility
    vascular occlusion
    hemiplegia
    osteoarthritis
    herpes zoster

ischemic contractures
    (sensory loss in fingers)
    tight plaster cast application

polyarteritis nodosa

polyneuritis
    carcinoma of lung
    Hodgkin's disease
    pregnancy
    gastric carcinoma
    reticuloses
    diabetes mellitus
    chemical neuritis
        antimony, benzene, bismuth, carbon tetrachloride, heavy
        metals, alcohol, arsenic, lead, gold, emetine
    ischemic neuropathy
    vitamin B deficiency
    atheromata
    arteriosclerosis
    embolic

carpodigital (carpopedal spasm) tetany
    hypoparathyroidism
    hyperventilation
    uremia
    nephritis
    nephrosis
    rickets
    sprue
    malabsorption syndrome
    pregnancy
    lactation
    osteomalacia
    protracted vomiting
    pyloric obstruction
    alkali poisoning
    chemical toxicity
        morphine, lead, alcohol

tremor
    parkinsonism
    familial disorder
    hypoglycemia
    hyperthyroidism
    Wilson's disease (hepatolenticular degeneration)
    anxiety

tremor (*continued*)
  ataxia (frontal lobe lesions)
  athetosis
  alcoholism, narcotic addiction
  multiple sclerosis
  chorea (Sydenham's, Huntingdon's)
  neurasthenia
  senility
  cerebellar lesions
  occupational neuroses
  hepatic coma
  posthepatitic disorder
  paresis
  cold, fatigue
  lesions of red nucleus
  toxicity (heavy metals, barbiturates)

COLOR CHANGES IN THE HAND

cyanosis
  congestive heart failure
  Raynaud's phenomenon
    polyarteritis nodosa
    Buerger's disease
    scleroderma
    dermatomyositis
    systemic lupus erythematosus
    arteriosclerosis
    cervical rib
    tumors or aneurysms encroaching on the brachial plexus
  polycythemia
  obliterative vascular disease
    scalenus anticus and related syndromes
    ball valve thrombus
  syringomyelia (Morvan's disease)
  systemic lupus erythematosus
  dermatomyositis
  drug effects
    acetanilid
    Coumadin ("purple toes and fingers")
    phenolphthalein
  acrocyanosis (cold, wet, swollen hand)
  congenital heart disease
  arteriovenous aneurysm

cyanosis (*continued*)
    myxedema
    hemosiderin deposits in congestive heart failure in children
    cor pulmonale
    scalenus anticus syndrome

pallor
    anemia
    aortic insufficiency ("paradoxic pallor")
    Raynaud's phenomenon sequence
    vasospasm—fingertips
        tobacco
        anxiety
        vasomotor instability

rubor
    pellagra (dorsum)
    polycythemia
    systemic lupus erythematosus (fingertips)
    dermatomyositis
    erythromelalgia
        (see causes under "increased temperature")
    pink disease (acrodynia, Swift's disease, erythroedema)
    lymphocytic leukemia ("l'homme rouge")

pigmentation overlying the veins of the dorsum
    Hodgkin's disease

diffuse melanosis
    Addison's disease (black freckles)
    melanosarcoma

slate-gray pigmentation
    argyria

yellow palms
    pernicious anemia
    carotinemia
    laborer's callus

depigmentation
    vitiligo
    pinta
    postdermatitic
    scleroderma
    dermatomyositis

purpuric spots
    Osler's disease (familial hemorrhagic telangiectasia)
    Peutz-Jegher's syndrome
    subacute bacterial endocarditis
    thrombocytopenic purpura
    blood dyscrasias

SUBUNGUAL HEMORRHAGES

Rendu-Osler-Weber's (familial hemorrhagic telangiectasia)

rheumatic fever

subacute bacterial endocarditis

trichiniasis

blood dyscrasias associated with bleeding tendency

scurvy

PHYSICAL FINDINGS IN THE PALM

Dupuytren's contracture
    diabetes mellitus
    epilepsy
    cirrhosis
    Raynaud's disease
    scalenus anticus syndrome
    postmyocardial infarction
    syringomyelia
    normal persons

xanthomata
    familial disorder
    hypercholesterolemia
    diabetes mellitus
    nephrosis
    biliary cirrhosis
    chronic pancreatitis
    von Gierke's disease
    cobaltous chloride
    myxedema
    Hand-Christian-Schüller disease
    Gaucher's disease
    Niemann-Pick's disease

palmar erythema
    hepatic cirrhosis ("liver palms")
    pregnancy

palmar erythema (*continued*)
  alcoholism
  mitral insufficiency
  rheumatoid arthritis
  polycythemia
  diabetes mellitus
  tuberculosis (acroerythrosis)
  vitamin B deficiency
  hyperestrogenism
  beriberi
  shoulder-hand syndrome
  arsenical toxicity
  3–5 percent of normal persons

pain
  burning sensations in hookworm infestation
  alcoholic neuritis
  neuritis from any cause
  carpal tunnel syndrome (see median nerve)

unusual formation or color of palmar creases
  single transverse crease
    mongolian idiocy
    congenital sclerodactyly
  blue creases
    generalized purpura
  pale, silvery or white creases
    anemia (hemoglobin below 7 Gm./100 ml.)
  dark brown or black creases
    Addison's disease
  displacement of triradii (see "Dermatoglyphics"–Chapter 9)
    certain congenital cardiac malformations

petechiae
  blood dyscrasias
  thrombocytopenic purpura
  subacute bacterial endocarditis
  scurvy
  vitamin deficiency
  premenstrual

Janeway lesion
  subacute bacterial endocarditis

Osler's nodes
  subacute bacterial endocarditis

callus
> (see "Occupational Effects in the Hand," p. 148)
> (absence of callus in epidermolysis bullosa)

TEMPERATURE CHANGES IN THE HAND

increased:
- arteriovenous aneurysm (unilateral finding)
- aneurysm
- hyperthyroidism
- fever
- hypermetabolic states
    - pontine hemorrhage
- environmental heat
- Paget's disease of bone
- erythromelalgia (primary or secondary)
    - hypertensive cardiovascular disease
    - gout
    - diabetes mellitus
    - rheumatoid arthritis
    - arteriosclerosis
    - polycythemia

decreased:
- shock
- hypothyroidism
- agonal hand
- arterial occlusion
- ischemic contracture
- syringomyelia
- scleroderma
- dermatomyositis
- systemic lupus erythematosus
- Raynaud's phenomenon
- environmental cold
- neurasthenia
- normal persons
- peripheral vascular diseases
    - embolus
    - thromboangiitis obliterans
    - scalenus anticus and related syndromes
    - pulmonary hypertension
- acrocyanosis

CAPILLARY PULSATIONS OF FINGERTIP AND NAIL BED (QUINCKE PULSE)

aortic insufficiency

hyperthyroidism

high-output cardiac failure

anemia

high fevers

INOCULATED INFECTIOUS DISEASES WHICH PRODUCE CHANCRE-LIKE LESIONS ON THE HAND

sporotrichosis

anthrax

actinomycosis

tuberculosis

syphilis

coccidiomycosis

tularemia

leishmaniasis

blastomycosis

References

PREFACE

BEAN, W. B.: Circulation 8:117 (July) 1953.

BEHRMAN, H. T.: Dermatologic Clues to Internal Disease. Grune & Stratton, Inc., New York, 1947.

CARR, J. B.: The Life of Sir Arthur Conan Doyle. Harper & Brothers, New York, 1949.

DANIEL, T. B.: Role of Hand in Physical Diagnosis. J. Bowman Gray School Med. 2:23, 1944.

WEINER, K.: Skin Manifestations of Internal Disorders. C. V. Mosby Co., St. Louis, 1947.

DISORDERS OF THE ENDOCRINE SYSTEM

FISCHER, F. J., AND VAN DEMARK, R. E.: J. Bone Joint Surg. (Brit.) 27B:145 (Jan.) 1945.

GREENE, R.: Proc. Roy. Soc. Med. 44:155 (Oct.) 1950.

HADDAD, HECKEL M., AND WILKINS, LAWSON: Pediatrics 23:885 (May) 1959.

LISSER, H., AND ESCAMILLA, R. F.: Atlas of Clinical Endocrinology, 2nd ed. C. V. Mosby Co., St. Louis, 1962.

RAY, ESTEN W., AND GARDNER, LYTT: Pediatrics 23:520 (Mar.) 1959.

SIMPSON, S. L.: Major Endocrine Disorders, 3rd ed. Oxford University Press, Inc., 1959.

UHR, N., AND BEZAHLER, H. B.: Ann. Intern. Med. 54:443 (Mar.) 1961.

WERNER, A. A.: Endocrinology, 2nd ed. Lea & Febiger, Philadelphia, 1942.

WILLIAMS, R. H. (ed.): Textbook of Endocrinology, 3rd ed. W. B. Saunders Co., Philadelphia, 1962.

DISORDERS OF CONNECTIVE TISSUE

BREWERTON, D. A.: Ann. Rheum. Dis. 16:183 (June) 1958.

BUNNELL, S.: Surgery of the Hand, 3rd ed. J. B. Lippincott Co., Philadelphia, 1956.

CONKLIN, J. E., AND WHITE, W. L.: Surg. Clin. N. Amer. 40:531 (Apr.) 1960.

CRAIN, DARRELL C.: J.A.M.A. 170:795 (June 13) 1959.

GOLDEN, RICHARD, AND LAKIN, H.: New Eng. J. Med. 260:797 (Nov.) 1959.

HOLLANDER, J. L.: Comroe's Arthritis and Allied Conditions, 6th ed. Lea & Febiger, Philadelphia, 1960.

KILLIP, T., III, AND HOLMQUIST, N. D.: Ann. Intern. Med. 54:431 (Mar.) 1961.

LEITNER, S. M.: Der Morbus Benier-Boeck-Schaumann. Grune & Stratton, Inc., New York, 1949.

MAJOR, R. H., AND DELP, M. H.: Physical Diagnosis, 6th ed. W. B. Saunders Co., Philadelphia, 1962.

MONTGOMERY, M. M., et al.: Ann. Intern. Med. 51:105 (July) 1959.

NAKAMURA, T., AND AUERBACH, S. H.: J. Tenn. Med. Assn. 52:80 (Mar.) 1959.

PEARSON, CARL M.: Bull. Rheum. Dis. 12:269 (Feb.) 1962.

Primer on the Rheumatic Diseases: J.A.M.A. 171:1345, 1959.

SINCLAIR, R. J. G.: Bull. Rheum. Dis. 8:153 (Jan.) 1958.

STEIN, G. N., ISRAEL, H. L., AND SONES, M. A.: Arch. Intern. Med. 97:532 (May) 1956.

STEINBROCKER, O., AND ARGYROS, T. G.: Med. Clin. N. Amer. 42:75 (Nov.) 1958.

THIRTEENTH RHEUMATISM REVIEW: Ann. Intern. Med. 58:173 (Dec.) 1960.

WAKEFIELD, A. R.: Surg. Clin. N. Amer. 40:483 (Apr.) 1960.

WEGMAN, T.: Munchen. Med. Wschr. 102:40, 1926-29.

WOLFE, S. J., SUMMERSKILL, W. H. J., AND DAVIDSON, C. S.: New Eng. J. Med. 255:559 (Sept. 20) 1956.

DISEASES OF THE NERVOUS SYSTEM

BAKWIN, H., AND BAKWIN, R. M.: Clinical Management of Behavior Disorders in Children, 2nd ed. W. B. Saunders Co., Philadelphia, 1960.

BUTTERWORTH, T., AND BOWER, J. R.: Penn. Med. J. 62:201 (Feb.) 1959.

CROSS, R. L., DODDS, M. E., AND KNIGHTS, E. M.: Surgery 46:1135 (Dec.) 1959.

ELLIOTT, F. A., HUGHES, B., AND TURNER, J. W. A.: Clinical Neurology. Paul B. Hoeber, Inc., New York, 1953.

FAY, T.: J.A.M.A. 155:729 (June 19) 1954.

MILLICHAP, J. G., MILLER, R. H., AND BACKUS, R. E.: J.A.M.A. 179:589 (Feb.) 1962.

PENROSE, L. S.: The Biology of Mental Defect, 2nd ed. Grune and Stratton, Inc., New York, 1954.

WECHSLER, I.: A Textbook of Clinical Neurology, 9th ed. W. B. Saunders Co., Philadelphia, 1963.

WOLFF, C.: The Hand in Psychological Diagnosis. Methuen & Co., Ltd., London, 1951.

DISEASES OF THE CARDIOVASCULAR SYSTEM

ABRAMSON, DAVID I.: Diagnosis and Treatment of Peripheral Vascular Disorders. Hoeber-Harper, New York, 1956, pp. 185, 370.

ALLEN, E. V., BARKER, N. W., AND HINES, E. A., JR.: Peripheral Vascular Diseases, 3rd ed. W. B. Saunders Co., Philadelphia, 1962.

Allen, E. V., and Brown, G. E.: Amer. J. Med. Sci. 183:187 (Feb.) 1932.
Chase, R. A.: Surg. Clin. N. Amer. 40:471 (Apr.) 1960.
deTakats, G., and Fowler, E. F.: J.A.M.A. 179:1 (Jan. 6) 1962.
Duff, R. D.: Brit. Med. J. 2:974 (Oct. 27) 1956.
Goldsmith, G. A., and Brown, G. E.: Amer. J. Med. Sci. 189:819, 1935.
Holling, H. E., and Brodley, R. S.: J.A.M.A. 178:977 (Dec. 3) 1961.
Osler, William: Lectures on Angina Pectoris and Allied State. Appleton, New York, 1897, p. 50.
Shapiro, E., Lipkis, M. L., and Kahn, J.: Amer. J. Med. Sci. 214:288 (Sept.) 1947.
Silverman, J. J., and Bernstein, A.: J.A.M.A. 158:821 (July 9) 1955.
Silverman, J. J., and Littman, D. S.: New Eng. J. Med. 249:839 (Nov. 19) 1953.
Terry, R. B.: Lancet 1:757 (Apr. 10) 1954; 2:842 (Oct. 23) 1954.

DISORDERS OF METABOLISM

Bauer, and Klemperer: In Duncan, G. G. (ed.): Diseases of Metabolism, 4th ed. W. B. Saunders Co., Philadelphia, 1959.
Bearn, A. G., and McKusick, V. A.: J.A.M.A. 166:93 (Feb. 22) 1958.
Benemid: A Review of the Nature and Treatment of Gout. Merck, Sharp & Dohme, Philadelphia, 1956.
Boland, E. W.: World-Wide Abstracts (Jan.) 1950, p. 15.
Caplan, R. M., and Curtis, A. C.: J.A.M.A. 176:859 (June 10) 1961.
Lorincz, A. L., Malkinson, F. D., and Rothman, S.: Med. Clin. N. Amer. 44:249 (Jan.) 1960.
Ormsby, O. S., and Montgomery, H.: Diseases of the Skin, 8th ed. Lea & Febiger, Philadelphia, 1954.
Stanbury, J. B., Wyngaarden, J. B., and Fredrickson, D. S.: The Metabolic Basis of Inherited Disease, McGraw-Hill, Toronto, Canada, 1960.
Talbott, J. H.: Med. Sc. (July 10) 1959, p. 23.
Wiener, K.: Systemic Associations and Treatment of Skin Diseases. C. V. Mosby Co., St. Louis, 1955.

MISCELLANEOUS DISORDERS INVOLVING THE HAND

Bandler, M.: Gastroenterology 38:641 (Apr.) 1960.
Banyai, A. L., and Hirsh, L. H.: Urol. & Cutan. Rev. 50:282, 1946.
Bean, W. B.: Circulation 8:117 (July) 1953.
Bean, W. B.: Vascular Spiders and Related Lesions of the Skin. Charles C Thomas, Springfield, Illinois, 1958.
Blank, H., and Rake, G.: Viral and Rickettsial Diseases of the Skin, Eye and Mucous Membranes of Man. Little, Brown and Co., Boston, 1955.
Delman, A. J., Porush, J. G., and Schwartz, A. D.: Ann. Intern. Med. 55:471 (Sept.) 1961.
Feder, W., and Auerbach, R.: Ann. Intern. Med. 55:911 (Dec.) 1961.
Flatt, A. E.: Geriatrics 15:733 (Nov.) 1960.
Gaisford, J. C.: Surg. Clin. N. Amer. 40:549 (Apr.) 1960.
Manley, K. A., and Skyring, A. P.: Arch. Intern. Med. 107:183 (Feb.) 1961.

RICHARDSON, J. A., JR., AND DIDDAM, A. C.: Arch. Intern. Med. 109:186 (Feb.) 1962.

RONCHESE, F.: A.M.A. Arch. Derm. & Syph. 63:565 (May) 1951.

SCHWARTZ, L., TULIPAN, L., AND BIRMINGHAM, D. J.: Occupational Diseases of the Skin, 3rd ed. Lea & Febiger, Philadelphia, 1957.

SILVERSTEIN, E.: J. Lab. Clin. Med. 47:513 (Apr.) 1956.

WALSH, E. N., AND BECKER, S. W.: Arch. Derm. Syph. 44:616 (Oct.) 1941.

WIENER, K.: Med. Clin. N. Amer. 43:689 (May) 1959.

WINTROBE, M. M.: Clinical Hematology, 5th ed. Lea & Febiger, Philadelphia, 1961.

INFECTIONS OF THE HAND

DOWNING, J. G.: Cutaneous Manifestations of Systemic Diseases. Charles C Thomas, Springfield, Illinois, 1954.

GRESHAM, G. A., AND PHEAR, D. N.: Amer. J. Med. 23:671 (Oct.) 1957.

HAHN, A. G.: Am. Rev. Tuberc. 20:876, 1929.

RIORDAN, D. C.: J. Bone Joint Surg. 42-A:661 (June) 1960.

SUTTON, R. L., JR.: Diseases of the Skin, 11th ed. C. V. Mosby Co., St. Louis, 1956.

DISEASES OF THE NAILS

MUEHRCKE, R. C., Brit. M. J. 1:1327 (June 9) 1956.

SIBINGA, M. S.: Pediatrics 24:225 (Aug.) 1959.

WHITE, C. J.: Ciba Clin. Symp. Vol. 2, No. 5 (May-June) 1950.

DERMATOGLYPHICS

CUMMINS, H., AND MIDLO, C.: Fingerprints, Palms and Soles. Blakiston Div., McGraw-Hill Book Co., Inc., New York, 1943.

HALE, A. R., PHILLIPS, J. H., AND BURCH, G. E.: J.A.M.A. 176:41 (Apr.) 1961.

RAPHAEL, T., AND RAPHAEL, L. G.: J.A.M.A. 180:215 (Apr. 21) 1962.

RONCHESE, F.: Occupational Marks and Other Physical Signs: A Guide to Personal Identification. Grune & Stratton, Inc., New York, 1948.

Index

Page numbers in *italics* refer to illustrations.

Palmar erythema (*Cont.*)
  in shoulder-hand syndrome, 128
Palsy, cerebral, 13
Pancoast tumor, 35, 197
Pancreatitis, chronic, hyperlipemia in, 121
Panniculitis, febrile, shoulder-hand syndrome in, 35
Paralysis
  general, 71
  median nerve, 75, *76*
  radial nerve, *76*, 77
  ulnar nerve, 77, *78*
Paralysis agitans, 66
Parasitic infestation, clubbing of fingers in, 107
Paronychia in sarcoidosis, 50
Pellagra, *118*, 119
Pemphigus, butcher's, 152
Periarteritis nodosa, 97
Peripheral vascular disease, Raynaud's phenomenon in, 97, 169
Perspiration
  in anxiety states, 7
  in hyperthyroidism, 7
  in nerve injury, 63
Petechia, 137
  in subacute bacterial endocarditis, 94
Peutz-Jegher syndrome, *140*, 141
Peyronie's disease, Dupuytren's contracture in, 38
Photosensitivity
  in porphyria, 115
  in systemic lupus erythematosus, 43
Physical findings in the hand, outline of, 193-204
Pigmentation
  in Addison's disease, 11
  in arsenical toxicity, 156
  in hand-biting, 143, 175
  in hypoparathyroidism, 15
  in leprosy, 171
  in pellagra, 119
  in Peutz-Jegher syndrome, *140*
  in pinta, *162*
  in Raynaud's phenomenon, 102
  in scleroderma, *39*, 41
  in tuberculous verrucosa cutis, 163
Pink disease, 87
Pinta, *162*
Pituitary infantilism, 5
Pituitary insufficiency, 3
Pituitary obesity, 5, *6*
Plummer-Vinson's syndrome, 139
Polyarthritis in rubella, 171
Polycythemia, 107, 139, *176*
  cyanosis in, 175
Polycythemia vera, Raynaud's phenomenon in, 102
Polydactyly, 89, 107, 142, 157
Polymyositis, 41
Polyp of intestine, in Peutz-Jegher syndrome, 141
Porphyria, 115, *116*
Pregnancy, palmar erythema in, 128

Pruritus
  in arsenical toxicity, 156
  in pink disease, 87
  in xanthoma, 113
Pseudohypoparathyroidism, 16
Pseudopseudohypoparathyroidism, 16
Pseudoxanthoma elasticum, 52, *57*
Psoriasis, 30-33
  arthritis in, *31, 32*
  pitted nails in, *31, 32*
  skin rash in, 30
Pterygium
  in cretinism, 13
  in dermatomyositis, 43
Pulmonary abscess, osteoarthropathy in, 108
Pulmonary hypertension, Raynaud's phenomenon in, 102
Pulmonary hypertrophic osteoarthropathy, 108
Pulmonic cysts, *109*
Purpura, *136*, 137
  in diabetes mellitus, 113
  in senility, 133, 137
  in subacute bacterial endocarditis, 94
Pustule, malignant, *164*, 165

Quincke-pulse, 95, 203

Radiologist's hand, *153*, 155
Raynaud's disease and phenomenon, 100, *101, 168*
  clubbed fingers in, 107
  in dermatomyositis, 43
  edema of hand in, 131
  in peripheral vascular disease, 97, 169
  in pulmonary hypertension, 102
  in scalenus anticus and related syndromes, 96
  in scleroderma, 41
  in systemic lupus erythematosus, 45
Reiter's syndrome, 50, *51*
Rendu-Osler-Weber disease (hereditary hemorrhagic telangiectasia), *134*, 135
Rheumatic fever, fingernail changes in, 91
Rheumatoid arthritis, 22-30
  arteritis in, *29*
  dislocation of tendons in, *24*
  "opera-glass hand," 27
  palmar erythema in, 22, 128
  psoriasis in, *31, 32*
  rheumatoid nodules in, 27
  synovial cysts in, *25, 28*, 30
  ulnar deviation in, *25*, 27
Rib, cervical, 100
  gangrene of fingerprints in, 169
Rickets, 117
Roentgen irradiation, effect of, *153*, 155
Rubella, 171

Sarcoidosis, 50
  arthropathy in, *48*
  paronychia in, 50

"He who wants to know man must look upon him as a whole and not as a patched-up piece of work. If he finds a part of the human body diseased, he must look for the causes which produce disease, and not merely treat the external effects."

PARACELSUS (16TH CENTURY)